DEAFNESS

- AND HOW TO SURVIVE!

Olivia Lee

IAN HENRY PUBLICATIONS
EMPIRE PUBLISHING SERVICE

ISBN 0 86025 541 7 (U.K.)
1 58690 018 8 (U.S.A.)

Library of Congress Cataloging-in-Publication Data

Lee, Olivia

Deafness – and how to survive! / Olivia Lee
1 Deafness. 2. Deafness in children. I. Title
RF290.L42 2006
617.8-dc22

Published by
Ian Henry Publications, Ltd.
20 Park Drive, Romford, Essex RM1 4LH
in association with
Empire Publishing Service
P O Box 1344, Studio City, California 91604
and printed by
Progress Press Co., Ltd.
Strickland House, 341 St Paul Street, Valletta, Malta

CHAPTERS

INTRODUCTION

When I first thought about writing a book on the problems of being deaf I wanted to call it *Why Don't They Listen?* but I felt that would make it sound too much like the by-product of some well-meaning agony column! Even so, it really is very frustrating for a deaf person when people refuse to listen to a simple plea to speak more clearly.

It is equally difficult for the genuinely concerned hearing person to know how best to help without denting those things called pride and independence of spirit. Nobody other than fashion slaves wishes to go around wearing a large label on their backs, least of all one that bears the message:

WARNING! THIS PERSON IS DEAF!

That is just asking to become a target practice spot for the less intelligent members of our society.

So, what should be done?

In this book I have attempted to tackle the problem by dealing with both points of view; those who are deaf, or hearing-impaired, and those whose good hearing makes it difficult or even impossible to imagine what the difficulties are.

Excellent books have already been written on topics such as the causes of deafness and their treatments, the wide range of technical aids available, and help with education and learning difficulties, to name just a few. Just one visit to the local library or the audiology clinic to glance along the bookshelf or information rack set aside for this kind of literature will confirm this. The reading materials available are ideal for looking at particular topics in greater detail but there appears to be no one book which includes all of these issues and more. It is one of the aims of this book to rectify that situation.

A large number of voluntary organisations, both national and regional, have been set up over the years to address the problems relating to deafness and details of many of them can be found throughout and at the end of this book. They are much used by the members of the deaf and hard-of-hearing community but are usually the last sort of people a hearing person would normally think of to seek out help.

For that reason I would like to see this book read by all those who come into regular contact with members of the public and the community at large, as part of their basic work or career training.

I have endeavoured to treat the subject with humour wherever it is possible; the distinctive feature of most deaf people is their ability to laugh at themselves and their situation. They have to in order to survive!

Olivia Lee

Chelmsford, England

CHAPTER ONE

WHAT IS DEAFNESS?

If you look in a dictionary you will see that it is likely to define the word deaf as being wholly or partly without hearing. It will probably go on to tell you that it can also mean being insensitive to harmony or rhythm. Further definitions, used in combination with other words to express different situations include being uncompliant, unresponsive or to simply ignore. And those are only the politest expressions!

So what does it mean to be deaf?

Let us put aside the dictionary and consider the question in real terms.

It means that for any child or adult who is deaf it is a daily battle to keep pace with those in the hearing world.

For a start, their outward appearances are against them! At first sight they usually look no different from any other member of the human race, unless they are unfortunate enough to have some kind of additional physical or second sensory disability such as blindness. If they are lucky, they will have two legs, two arms, a body to which these are attached, a head and face, and a shell-like appendage to each side of the head which are called ears.

So, if they have ears then surely they must be able to hear? Ha!

'Why not?' do you ask?

Simple. There is far more to the workings of the ear than first meets the eye.

The external bit you see is specially shaped for gathering sound. Who has never come across the expression, *a word in your shell-like ear*?

How many times have you watched an animal twitch or turn its ears to listen to something and so track down the direction from which the sound comes? The larger and more mobile the ears, the better.

There are a few unusual humans who can waggle their earflaps, usually for a party piece, but in general our ears stay in a fixed position. This puts us way down in the hearing ability league compared with the rest of the animal world. True, it is a scientific fact that our external ears continue to grow throughout our lives - as if to compensate for the gradual hearing loss which happens to most of us as time goes by.

So why should our hearing deteriorate?

Well, why not? Young footballers occasionally need to have operations to their knees, athletes damage tendons and ligaments in their legs, computer keyboard operators damage fingers and wrists - the list is endless. Each is an example of a deteriorating physical condition through excessive or too much repetitive use, proof that we do not have to wait until we grow old for things to go wrong with our bodies or our senses.

So how can we compare these with something that is invisible, such as hearing loss?

There are many instances. Here we will look at what is likely to happen to the young child, born with normal hearing, from the time he or she begins experiencing life through to mature adulthood.

Right from the start we are bombarded with noise of all kinds: traffic, music, domestic power tools, roadworks and heavy machinery, to name but a few. And where is the child when all this is going on? He has little choice but to be constantly on the receiving end - children are far more capable of absorbing loud noises that they learn to tolerate. And that is where the danger lies. It is during this period that the most damage is likely to be done to our hearing ability. Only when we grow older do harsh or excessive sounds become painful to tolerate.

Through the media we are made aware of the increasing number of young people who are becoming deaf or deafened at a prematurely early age. Why? Why not, when you consider their lifestyles. There can be few who do not enjoy listening to the latest trends in popular music, and with the sound volume turned at full blast! Nothing too much wrong with that if they listen to it only for short periods but the modern trend is to wear earplugs or headphones linked to personal stereo systems. When these are kept running in this manner for hour after hour, this is just asking for trouble.

What happens when a young teenager arrives at his place of work the morning after spending mind-blowing hours using this ear-blasting form of entertainment? Apart from being unable to concentrate on anything useful, his or her ears will be ringing and buzzing a tune all to themselves. If he works in an office he is likely to waste much time trying to answer telephones that are not actually ringing; if in a supermarket the bleeping of cash registers will merge with his or her own personal orchestra; and on a building site or in a factory the added noise of heavy powered machinery could make him think he had wandered into a theme park nightmare!

So, why should excessive sound damage the hearing?

To answer that we first need to ask ourselves - what is sound?

Think about what happens when a door is slammed shut. Apart from the probable unpleasant reason for it being slammed in the first place, you will feel a bit of a draught! You may feel the walls or floor shaking from the impact and you will almost certainly feel pain or discomfort in your ears and head as the noise hits you. That simple but upsetting action of slamming will have brought about changes in the air pressure around you known as sound waves.

Those hard-hitting vibrations can also make you feel physically ill for a while, sometimes so much so that you may feel giddy and want to lie down. And this is in addition to the circumstances that brought about the action in the first place.

So what did happen when the sound waves reached the ear? Well, for a start, they shot straight along the ear passage at a fair old speed, hitting the ear-drum with a wallop! Enough to make your head spin - just like when any drum is struck.

The impact set off a chain reaction from the three tiny bones positioned just behind the ear-drum. These were ready and waiting to transmit the vibrations onwards to the fluid-filled cavity of the inner ear. Once inside the cavity they then moved through the fluid, rather as ripples move across a pond surface, activating the endings of the hearing nerve that is linked directly to the brain. It is when the frequency of these vibrations becomes excessive that the nerve endings are damaged, leading to lasting hearing loss. Unlike skin, nerve fibres do not normally grow again.

How come all this might make us feel sick and giddy? In this instance the blame lies in that disturbance of the inner ear. Within that cavity are three semi-circular canals that link to a second nerve leading directly to the brain. This nerve interprets the messages being sent to instruct the body on how to stay upright. If those canals are disturbed or damaged too much then incorrect signals will be received - the kind that can suddenly send you flat on your back or similar uncomfortable or painful position!

All this is only a very simplified description of how the ear works but it should go some way to helping to understand how our hearing can be lost, whether it be temporary or permanent.

There are two main types of deafness: conductive, and sensori-neural or nerve deafness. The last named is also known as perceptive deafness.

Conductive deafness can occur when the conduction of sound on its way to the inner ear is reduced as a result of damage to the ear-drum or to the chain of small bones in the middle ear. These can usually be cured or improved upon by drugs or surgery.

It can also result from a simple blockage of the ear canal from wax or from water, as when swimming or washing our hair. We can easily shake out excess water but wax is a more solid substance, as any inquisitive child will quickly discover. Parental reaction to a demonstration of this kind of discovery is usually one of disapproval, if not sheer disgust.

The purpose of the wax is to protect the inner cavities of the ear from any unwanted and damaging particles of dust or grit which may enter through the external ear passage. When larger particles, like the kind of small objects so beloved of young children, are poked and wedged into ears, it will be panic stations! The wax will build up into a large blob in the attempt to push out any foreign object. The result is partial or complete deafness. Fortunately medical staff are trained to remove this kind of obstruction and so there should be no need for tears at bedtime, at least not until the next crisis.

At the base of the middle ear there is a small tube or canal which leads downward to the cavity linking the nose and throat. This tube opens and closes under certain conditions to maintain an even air pressure within the cavity. Normally it is kept closed but it opens each time we swallow. Should this pressure become uneven, for whatever reason, the result would be injury to the ear and probable permanent deafness. Think about what happens when you are suffering from a heavy cold. What with excessive fluid build-up and the body's constant attempts to clear it away through sneezing, nose-clearing or coughing, the air pressure in the cavity becomes so badly affected that it is almost impossible to hear clearly. Thankfully this is a situation which usually rights itself after a few days.

A more permanent form of conductive deafness can be caused by disease processes that bring about physical changes in the middle ear or in the bones around its labyrinth, such as a gradual overgrowth of bone.

Sensori-neural (nerve) deafness is generally due to damage to or destruction of the nerve fibres and endings of the auditory (hearing) nerve. In the past this has been almost impossible to treat but advances are being made to improve on this kind of hearing loss.

Damage to the nerve endings may be caused through illnesses such as measles, mumps, or spinal meningitis, or if the mother was ill with German measles (Rubella) during pregnancy. Progressive conditions, such as Menière's, will eventually affect the hearing as well as the sense of balance. Taking certain drugs may bring about changes in the auditory nerve or in the brain centre of hearing. The latter can also happen when the brain is unexpectedly deprived of its vital supply of oxygen.

A child may be born deaf as the result of some defect in the development of the inner ear or may go deaf in infancy through one of the childhood illnesses referred to above. Even a simple infection, which for one reason or another did not respond to treatment, may cause deafness.

There are also inherited diseases which cause progressive deafness, such as Usher's Syndrome which will also cause blindness during childhood and through into adulthood.

Increasing deafness in adulthood is much more difficult to cope with since more often than not it is combined with having to cope with additional physical or mental problems as well. This in turn will add to the stress of the situation, about more of which will be learnt in a later chapter.

Tinnitus is not a type of deafness but brief mention of it must be made here, as it is something that affects the majority of those who have hearing difficulties. It can also affect those with normal hearing.

The medical name, *tinnitus*, is given for what is generally described as noises in the ear or inside the head. It is certainly not a sign of madness although its victims, and sometimes their nearest and dearest, would be forgiven for thinking otherwise.

Think of what it is like trying to hear when you have a heavy cold and then try to imagine how someone with a normally poor level of hearing would cope both with understanding the spoken word and the additional aggravation of tinnitus. Fraught!

Those unintelligible noises, which really do come from within the body or head, can dominate external sounds and speech so much that they will create an almost intolerable situation. This will set up a vicious circle by causing more stress. There is little in the way of medication to relieve this distressing problem but much research has been made into ways of helping and professional advice is available on learning how to cope.

CHAPTER TWO

FAMILY SUPPORT

We all know how easy it is to want to lash out in anger when well-laid plans go badly wrong. Parents will despair when told there is something amiss with their new-born baby. A middle-aged couple, looking forward to having a few happy and healthy retirement years together, can have their hopes dashed by unexpected serious health problems. Teenagers about to start a new job or follow a long-term career path can be thrown off course by obstructive circumstances for which he or she had been unprepared. Sudden hearing loss, in fact, can happen to anyone at any age with traumatic effect when normal communication becomes impossible.

A natural reaction in any of these situations is to look around for someone to blame. The father of a child born with a congenital form of deafness may turn against the mother or he, or the mother, or both of them, may blame the medical staff whom they believed had allowed this to happen. Likewise there may be a similar reaction if an older child becomes deaf or deafened through illness or an accident. Interestingly enough the children themselves do not react in this way. It is not until they become much older that they begin to question their existence - and just about every other subject - a fact that is likely to test the patience of adults to the very limit.

After the period of blame comes the feeling of guilt. This is something that is experienced at all levels. A mother will feel guilty that such a thing has happened to her child and may well carry this as a personal cross to bear for the remainder of her life.

It will be of little comfort to her to have the adult-child quote the old saying that 'what you don't know about, you don't miss'. Quite the opposite may happen to the older person doing well in his job or career or for the middle-aged couple where so many things once taken for granted would be missed. The partner physically unaffected by deafness may feel guilty at being unable to cope with this changed situation. A teenager, on the other hand, would not begin to feel guilt over those first angry reactions until shown how to cope with and adapt to the situation.

By trying to understand some of the problems involved we can learn how to overcome them and then move onwards to improve the quality of life. Working together in mutual co-operation to achieve this can bring its own reward.

One of the most satisfying experiences any parent can have is hearing their child learn to talk. This may well, later on, drive them mad when the talking doesn't stop! Intelligible talk, however, is only produced as the result of patient and constant correction and by setting a good example in the first place. Something that is far easier said than done.

What happens when a newly fixed kitchen shelf collapses? Or someone discovers that the next-door's cat has just helped himself to a freshly cooked portion of chicken? Or worse, the fairy lights on the Christmas tree have fused for the umpteenth time? The list of dramas is endless but what does all this have to do with bringing up a deaf child? A lot more than you think.

What happens with our body language, our facial expressions, or other people's reactions in these situations? From the deaf child's viewpoint this will all look like one great big joke. The adult, in the heat of the moment, will assume the child is being deliberately naughty or cheeky and will start to shout back and pull bad-tempered looking faces. This will then frighten and upset the child and the situation can go full circle until it gets back to that state of blame and guilt. Unless, of course, you are one of those wonderful people who simply never get upset about anything?

In an example of what life can be like for our middle-aged couple visualise the scene where the husband has gone to his little workshop, be it in the house basement or the outdoor shed. Somehow the external door-latch to this drops down, locking him in. His wife, who is deaf, cannot hear him shouting and in any case is otherwise preoccupied reading a good book. Some two hours later when he reappears in the house she cannot understand why he is looking so angry. It is so difficult for her cope with lip-reading his teeth-clenching explanation of how he has broken or bent half his tool kit working to dismantle the door, the window, or the lock, or whatever, to set himself free.

In a situation like that blame and guilt are likely to follow in equal measure but at least this lady did not make matters worse by also accidentally locking her husband out of the house. A quick peek at Chapter 4 can give some hints on how this scenario might have been avoided in the first place.

Often the first time a deaf or deafened child may experience problems outside the secure world of the home unit is when mixing in a full-time education environment. If he is profoundly deaf then he will never have understood speech and will have developed mentally only through the use of the simplest forms of sign language and general observations. His schooling will need to be carried out at either a special needs school or a special needs unit at a local school. With the former there will be the additional trauma of being away from home and all things familiar for long periods. For the latter, realisation that most other children do not go around needing to wear hearing-aids can come as a shock. Experiencing for the first time the blunt questioning curiosity of those who have never before seen a hearing-aid or heard anyone speak in such a strange-sounding way compounds this. Unlike adults, children still have to learn how to ignore cruel-sounding jibes.

For the child or teenager whose deafness is progressive there is a two-fold problem. Apart from having to cope with their hearing loss they also have to learn to lip-read and to use one of the forms of sign language best suited to their needs. All this is in addition to getting through the education system with reasonable success and having to change to schools more suited to their level of deafness. Some young people will also have to cope with the additional problems of deteriorating eyesight or other disabilities.

At the other end of the age scale older people who lose their hearing in later life will gradually forget how words should be pronounced and how to make the right pitch of sound. Remember that few deaf people are actually dumb. In the cases of those, both young and old, who are fortunate to regain all or part of their hearing, for whatever reason, they will need specialist help with relearning how to speak normally.

There was a time, not so long ago, when the only help families could expect to receive in coping with raising a deaf child would have been from a very small band of more enlightened teachers, doctors and social workers. These days, thanks to the hard work of the founder members of the numerous charities formed to help out in this way, most families requiring specialist services are almost spoilt for choice. As a consequence of the persistence from those far-sighted people attitudes have changed enormously but there is still much room for improvement.

There comes a time when, for example, most teenagers want to be part of the big world outside. Away from the reassuring surroundings of home and the special education unit the scene can change dramatically. They want to look and dress the same and experience new things. It takes a brave lad to have his hair cut short almost to the point of baldness with nothing to hide the hearing aid resting over his ear. Yes, it lets the world know that he has to be spoken to clearly in order to be understood but few teenagers have enough confidence to show their deafness in this way. The strange thing about this is that they never seem to mind flaunting clumps of earrings and other strange-looking metal objects clipped or stapled into their ears, noses and other unthinkable places!

Girls have a far better time of it fashion-wise. An earlier generation had to constantly juggle with the problem of hiding cumbersome body-worn hearing aids linked by long leads to the ear. Low cut necklines in warmer weather or for social occasions were definitely out. So were tight-fitting tops since the large microphones that were clipped to underwear stood out prominently in a most embarrassing fashion. It was tempting to leave the hearing aid at home but the thought of missing out on all the gossip usually won the day.

In general, most teenagers get by in coping with building up their social lives and developing their adult character through the help and support of relatives and friends and from charities specialising in helping young people to improve their lives. Coping in a working environment, however, is another matter and this topic is covered in Chapters 5 and 6.

Society seems to adopt a quite different attitude towards any older person seen wearing a hearing aid, probably because the wearer usually has grey or greying hair. In the minds of the less well-informed, grey hair and hearing-aids conjure up a more conventional and acceptable image. And should that person also be carrying around a white stick, then so much the better. No wonder some of the recently deafened and still very independent minded older people insist on managing without a hearing-aid, to the exasperation of their long suffering families. Cantankerousness is an understatement where such free spirits are concerned, but who can blame them? While society persists in labelling all old people as frail and senile when they are merely deaf, or blind, or both, such well-meaning and supportive families will go on having their patience pushed to the very limits.

CHAPTER THREE

HEARING AIDS

For the person newly diagnosed as deaf a whole new world is opened up just waiting to be explored. It can either become a very exciting time or a miserable one depending upon how they approach it and the kind of support they have. Modern technology has advanced so much that there is little a deaf or deafblind person cannot achieve.

For all but the most profoundly deaf there is a comprehensive range of hearing aids designed to suit individual needs. However, it is important to remember that whether the aid is selected by an audiologist in the NHS (National Health Service) hearing aid department or offered by a registered private hearing aid dispenser, a hearing aid is no more than a sound amplifier.

But what a versatile tool it is! It has a simple on/off switch, a volume control, a tiny microphone for receiving sound, a tone control for adjusting to the best pitch of sound and most hearing-aids have a switch with a T position. This switch works in conjunction with an inductive coupler in the earpiece that can be used with the different types of assistive communication aids described in Chapter 4.

The most frequently used type of aid is that worn behind the ear but there are also the body-worn types, those that fit into the ear and spectacle aids. The latter two are not generally available through the NHS and are more expensive; the first because of the precisioning of its technical components within a correctly moulded ear fitting and the second because of the additional cost and fitting of prescription lenses, as well as the hearing-aid unit, within the spectacle frame.

Body-worn aids come in the form of a compact case, usually worn close to the chest when clipped on to clothing. A cord links this to the earphone that is connected to an ear-mould fitted into the ear. These aids are usually high-powered, but now that the high-powered behind-the-ear type of aid is widely available they are a less popular option. Nevertheless for those whose hands and fingers are disabled, for whatever reason, its larger sized controls are easier to use.

Anyone who has been diagnosed by an Ear Nose and Throat (ENT) specialist as having an inadequate level of hearing is entitled to be given one hearing-aid, free of charge, through the NHS. An audiologist in the Hearing-Aid department will assess the level of hearing loss by using an audiometer, an instrument that measures the quietest sounds that can be heard over a range of frequencies or different pitches. On the basis of that assessment a hearing-aid that is most suited to the type and degree of hearing loss will be selected.

The main problem with an audiogram test is that it only measures indoor hearing ability in an artificial environment. It is not an assessment of how hearing affects mobility or orientation, particularly out of doors where background noise such as traffic and general street noises will affect the deaf person's ability to communicate.

Another problem for the first time wearer is the physical strangeness of wearing a hearing-aid. It is important that the aid should fit comfortably over the ear and without causing concern that it is about to fall off. This is particularly noticeable by those who have to wear glasses as well but the solution is a simple one. Any qualified optician will be able to shape the arms of the spectacles to fit more closely behind the ear.

Many Hearing-Aid departments operate a follow up system to help the wearer to adjust to using the aid and to resolve any problems that might subsequently occur through its use.

For whatever reason a person chooses to buy a hearing-aid from a private dispenser they are strongly advised to go to one which is registered to do so, preferably one with a permanent office near to home. Special care has to be exercised in selecting and fitting any hearing-aid since the maximum sound pressure capability may impair the remaining hearing of the user. For that reason alone never allow others to wear your hearing aid.

Just as with buying any other expensive item, commonsense should prevail to see that the type of aid chosen is one that is going to give the best hearing advantage. The preferred type of aid should be tried out both in the quiet of the consulting room and in the normal, and usually far noisier and more distracting, environment of the home, and at work if applicable, before making the final decision to buy.

Prices are not quoted in this book for the simple reason that what may be correct now may not be so two or three years on. Many of the organisations named in the Helplist will be happy to give up-to-date information on prices and advise on the range of aids available. Some will be able to arrange demonstrations of these and other types of assistive aids. The latter can be used in addition to or instead of personally-worn hearing aids.

All hearing aids should be used in conjunction with a closely fitting ear-mould. If it is too loose then the full benefit of the sound enhancement produced by the hearing-aid will be lost. It will also result in a high pitched whistling that is likely to cause unpopularity with the neighbours, unless of course the wearer is living on a deserted island!

The ear-mould is made from an impression of the ear taken by an audiologist. Reputable private dispensers will do this but often at extra cost. The mould impressions are taken using a silicon putty, a painless experience. Any discomfort is likely to be purely imaginary, prompted by the brief slight pressure as a putty material is moulded into the hollow of the external ear. It is all over in less two minutes.

Gone are the days when first a wad of gauze was poked into the ear canal followed by warm, sometimes too warm, wax being poured into the outer ear, then the long wait for it to cool and set - with a stiff neck and a bruised 'good side' as a result. Pity the young, profoundly deaf, child who had to suffer both ears being assaulted in this way. For today's youngsters, accustomed to the rituals of hearing tests from the first weeks of independent life, such ear mould fitting sessions are all part and parcel of what for them is a normal way of life.

Anyone who has ever worn earrings for any length of time will testify that skin is sensitive to pain and discomfort. For this reason-ear moulds are made from a variety of materials selected for the best needs of the wearer. If the aid is going to be worn continuously throughout each waking day then the ear-mould has to be made of a flexible material, such as soft acrylic, in order to avoid a build-up of painful pressure against the ear.

For the first-time user a hard acrylic is used in making the mould. The same type of material is used for those with a moderate hearing loss who only need a hearing aid for occasional use. There are some less fortunate people who have skin that is sensitive or allergic to man-made materials. For them, ear-moulds are made from natural materials like silicone, coe or vulcanite. Silicone is also used when an ear-mould is required with a high-powered hearing-aid. That type of aid is usually worn almost continuously and the silicone material is a non-allergic alternative to soft acrylic.

Whichever type of mould is worn a little dab of Vaseline or light skin cream smeared over the surface of the ear hollow helps the mould to be slipped into place more easily and quickly. If only for this reason both the ear-mould and hearing-aid should be kept clean with a dry soft cloth and checked to see that there is no wax left behind in the ear-mould openings.

Hearing-aids function only when batteries are fitted and are supplied free with those aids provided by the NHS. The length of time they last depends on the size of the aid. Batteries for privately dispensed hearing-aids can be purchased from most stockists. Rechargeable ones, if they are the right size, may also be used but are far more expensive to buy.

There are several important things to remember about the care of batteries. It is recommended that the battery is removed from the hearing-aid at night, particularly if you are likely to forget to turn off the aid when no longer wearing it. The same rule applies when the aid is not going to be used for a length of time, such as during the period of getting used to wearing a hearing aid for the first time. If you do leave the battery in then try to remember to open the battery drawer to give the aid the chance to dry out.

Batteries are liable to run down without warning and so always carry a spare. Spent batteries may leak inside your hearing-aid, causing serious damage if not promptly removed. Never dispose of them in fire but discard in a place where small children or pet animals cannot reach them.

The hearing aid can be supplied with a tamper resistant battery drawer. This is strongly recommended for infants, small children and persons of mental incapacity.

New batteries should be kept separate in a cool dry place, and in the original packet to prevent shorting, using the oldest ones first. Never try to recharge a battery unless it is of the type designed for that purpose and always use batteries specified by the hearing aid specialist.

Last, but not least, always check medication before swallowing since batteries are small enough to be mistaken for pills. Sometimes we are too tired, or perhaps too unwell, to remember routine things but by making the extra effort unwanted accidents and damage to the hearing-aid can be avoided.

For those with poor hearing in both ears it can help to wear two hearing aids. After all, Nature designed us to have two ears to use. Young deaf children are provided with this facility to help with their general and educational development but this is not always the case for an adult. Those who do require or request a second hearing-aid are generally expected to purchase one through a private dispenser, unless they can prove that their work and therefore their living is being affected by this restriction. For some people that it is not a satisfactory situation.

An ideal hearing-aid would be one which offered all the benefits of normal hearing: the ability to hear speech against noisy backgrounds, to quickly adjust from quiet to noisy situations, to protect from any sudden intense sounds, to hear speech more clearly and follow whole sentences or more. A tall order but our scientists and technicians are getting there.

New digital programming techniques for developing sound processing systems are making such hearing-aids possible by converting sound into a series of numbers - language that the tiny computers used in them can understand. Most of them can cut out some kinds of background noise but it is worth remembering that there are some analogue aids designed to do this too. The technology involved with digital aids makes them more expensive to buy but in time the costs involved will come down.

The final part of this chapter has been reserved for the mention of technology using surgical operating techniques.

Cochlear implants or 'bionic ears' are devices capable of greatly improving the hearing of profoundly deaf people by inserting electrodes into the inner ear which stimulate its nerve cells. The electrodes are connected to a receiver linked to a microphone and speech processor that converts sounds into electrical signals. They enable children, born totally deaf, to hear sounds for the first time and to eventually interpret those sounds and speech as well as, if not better than, children who lost their hearing early in life. This operation is also available for adults although it is less successful in those who have never been able to hear than in those who had lost their hearing later in life after learning to speak.

The Symphonix Vibrant soundbridge is a microchip implant designed to bring sound vibrations directly to the middle ear, bypassing the ear-drum, and capable of increasing the sound volume without diminishing the clarity. The implant operation involves intricate and painstaking surgery and the external audio-processor used has to be tuned accurately to gain the best results.

As with so many operations there can be risks and, together with the necessary follow up treatment, are expensive. Further research work is continuing into the long-term advantages and disadvantages.

With all this progress being made it is possible that one day permanent deafness will have become a thing of the past.

CHAPTER FOUR

ASSISTIVE AIDS AND OTHER HELP

Laugh and the world laughs with you,
Weep, and you weep alone...

Ella Wheeler Wilcox, the author of these famous lines, could not possibly have foreseen how true those words would become for the wearers of hearing-aids.

How many times have users turned up the volume of the aid to catch the punch line of a joke being told then frantically turned it down again as the noise of the laughter that followed became unbearable, making them want to weep with the pain?

Nowadays it is possible to avoid such misery by taking advantage of the many assistive sound enhancement systems available which can be used in conjunction with, or even independent of, hearing aids. Designed to link directly with a microphone they minimise the kind of background noise that would otherwise cause so much distress.

Loop systems work by sending the required sound signal to a hearing aid. The concept is simple. A sound input to a loop amplifier attached to a loop of wire around a room transmits the sound source to the inbuilt receiver coil inside a hearing-aid or other suitable receiver. When the hearing-aid is switched from the M to the T position the user is free to move anywhere within that looped area and be able to listen to the sound source, such as a television or radio programme. To gain the most benefit some volume adjustment may be required when switching to the T position on the aid but this will not affect the level of sound volume being heard by other people in the room.

These systems can be used not only in domestic living rooms but can also be found in many public places such as churches, theatres, banks and railway stations. There are a few situations where it may not be satisfactory to install a loop system due to magnetic noise interference with the loop signals but these are few.

Battery powered portable personal loop systems, including those referred to as Conference Folders, allow the features of a fixed loop system to be used by an individual without the need to install a loop cable around the room. The user wears a small loop around the neck or alongside the hearing aid that is connected to the portable unit. For those who do not wish to wear a neck loop alternative ear loops are available. The disadvantage of these is that they are inclined to slip away from the ear at inconvenient moments. The easy portability of these personal systems offers the advantage of being able to use them in places like meeting room halls where an integrated permanent loop system has never been installed.

Infrared assistive listening systems are an alternative to loop systems. Mains-powered transmitters pick up the sound via a small microphone and send it to the receiver by means of an invisible infrared light. Rechargeable batteries power this receiver, in the form of either a lightweight headset or a neck loop. As with the loop system it allows the user to control the volume without disturbing others. It also has the advantage of no trailing wires and is compatible with most cinema and theatre equipment.

The range of portable systems has expanded enormously. Whatever may seem suitable at first sight should be tried out before purchasing, whenever possible, and so avoid any unnecessary expenditure. As mentioned in the previous chapter many of the organisations named in the Helplist will be happy to advise in greater detail. Quite often they are able to show sample products of the type of aids available.

For those with moderate hearing loss or who have chosen not to wear a hearing-aid for whatever reason, personal amplifying systems are also available for use without a hearing aid. These will work in exactly the same way as when a hearing aid is switched to the T position.

Not so long ago using a telephone would have been a nerve-wracking experience for any person classed as hard of hearing and a demoralising impossibility for the more severely deafened the deaf and the deafblind. Nowadays, the wonders of ever-advancing technology have created a range of telephones and computer software that have helped to break down many of the old sound barriers created by the hearing world. There are telephones with adjustable amplifiers, and a wide range of fixed line and portable textphones through which conversations can be typed out or spoken. For those less confident at typing from a keyboard faxphones are ideal for transmitting handwritten messages

Text-messaging through the widespread of digital mobile phones is another ideal way to communicate. Some include inductive loopsets that can be used by those who need to wear a hearing aid - the Nokia LPS-1 is one of them. They can be carried either around the neck or discreetly hidden under clothes. A built-in microphone allows for handfree operation to do other jobs, such as writing down information, while talking on the phone. They also have a vibrating battery option - useful for knowing when there is an incoming call!

Computer hardware and software technology now make it possible for a deafblind person to communicate through the help of Braille displays, speech synthesizers or large-character software.

For those hearing people needing to contact a deaf person by telephone a system known as Typetalk has been set up. This is a national telephone relay service developed by BT (British Telecom) and the RNID through which, with the help of their specially trained operators, telephone calls can be made and received between those who use ordinary telephones and those who can only use a textphone.

Through the use of computer hardware and software it has become possible to make and receive telephone calls using picture imaging. This breakthrough is of great benefit to those who use lip-reading or some form of sign language, or both, to assist in understanding the spoken word.

Fixed line telephones can be linked with a flashing light or an additional sound amplifier, or both, to warn of incoming calls. Door chimes, bedside alarm clocks, and baby monitoring alarms will alert the user in a similar way.

For the deafblind, fans can be operated when a doorbell is rung and Braille alarm clocks can be fitted with a special unit known as the Sentinel that can operate with a personal vibrator.

Personal pagers are designed to vibrate against the user when triggered by a signal from the sound source to which it is linked. There are complete personal paging systems that can be set up very simply and used to include fire or smoke detector alarms, burglar alarms and even car alarms. Obviously to buy a full system, and to allow for essential running costs such as battery replacements, would work out expensive but the confidence gained through being able to live a reasonably independent life is so rewarding.

The Teletext and subtitling system used with many television programmes is a boon for those who are too severely deaf to follow any sound commentary but until quite recently it had not been possible to record those subtitles using a video recorder. All that has changed. Now it is possible to enjoy commercially available videos made with subtitles by using a video caption-reader linked to the video recorder. The range of film titles to choose from includes not only the best, and sometimes the worst, but also those produced as educational aids to important subjects like fingerspelling and sign language presentation.

It is useful to know that under the provisions of Group 14 of Schedule 5 to the Value Added Tax Act 1983 many of these technical aids referred to can be purchased exclusive of V.A.T. if the user has to wear a hearing-aid or is registered as having a hearing loss.

Not everyone is able to take advantage of modern technology and there are some who will never feel comfortable with using it. For them the alternative is to make use of one or more of the many forms of manual communication such as sign language in various forms, signing, the deafblind manual alphabet, lip-reading, fingerspelling and use of interpreters.

British Sign Language is a language all of its own, used by those who were born severely or profoundly deaf or who became deaf before acquiring speech. Also used by members of the hearing community in regular contact with the deaf it is a rich and complex visual language with its own grammar and idioms. Just as with any national sign language, such as American Sign Language, it will vary from region to region.

Paget Gorman Signed Speech differs from this in that it provides an exact grammatical signed representation of spoken English. Children with speech and language disorders mainly use it.

Signed English uses signs from British Sign Language but with the addition of markers and generated signs, together with fingerspelling, to reproduce the components of grammatical English. It is intended for use with deaf and hard-of-hearing schoolchildren in order to develop reading and writing skills.

Gestuno Sign Language was created for use as a second language for international communication between deaf people.

Bliss Symbols are another means of international communication, created to use with children. They are of particular help to those with physical disabilities who are unable to otherwise communicate.

The Makaton Vocabulary provides a basic means of communication. It encourages language development in children with learning or communication difficulties and is of equal benefit to those with multiple disabilities.

Sign Supported English uses sign language, spoken English and fingerspelling in the same order as the spoken word. It is intended as a compromise between sign language and spoken English.

Cued Speech is compatible with both lip-reading and sign language. It uses simple hand shapes to represent the sounds of speech.

Fingerspelling is the deafblind manual alphabet using one sign for each letter. It can be spelt into either hand of the 'listener'.

The Deafblind Block Alphabet is an alternative method of fingerspelling where each letter of the alphabet is drawn out across the palm of the hand.

For some deaf people and hearing-aid users the easiest way to communicate is by Lip-reading. This will be referred to in more detail in later chapters.

Total Communication is an approach that may use any or all of the following: signing, finger-spelling, lip-reading, residual hearing and spoken language. It is widely used in teaching deaf children.

An Interpreter, in the context of this book, is any person who has undergone professional training in one or more of the communication skills described in this chapter. They play an important part in the lives of deaf and hearing people, giving them access to information in a variety of settings: attending conferences, courses, job interviews, Court, landmark ceremonies such as marriage, or even visits to the doctor or dentist. They are highly trained and are often able to give a deaf person the information in easier terms without changing the meaning of the words spoken. Interpreters have now made it possible for deaf people to enjoy the theatre.

Lip-speakers have a similar rôle to interpreters; they convey information to lip-readers without using their voice.

What happens when all this marvellous technology breaks down or there is no neighbour, family member or friend on hand to help?

There are Hearing Dogs for the deaf, specially trained to recognise and respond to a variety of sounds such as alarm clocks, door bells, telephones, and even oven-timers. And of course they can make first class companions!

CHAPTER FIVE

EDUCATION

Hearing and sight are the two senses through which we receive 95 per cent of all that we learn about the world around us. When these are absent or incomplete then other senses such as touch and smell have to be used to a much greater extent to compensate for those losses.

Our education begins the day we are born, some would argue that it starts long before then. Touch, from adult caring hands, is usually the first sense we experience and will play a large part in our early education. Through this sense we will discover people, objects of all shapes and sizes, fabrics and textures, plant life, insect life and animals. It is senses such as hearing, sight, or smell that inform us of anything that might endanger us were we to rely upon touch alone.

It is for this reason that for any child born without hearing or sight, or who loses one or the other or both at a later stage of development, priority has to be given to work out the best means of communication suited to its disability. To do this will require services specially designed to ensure that each child's development and education is built upon as surely as those with all of their senses, giving them an equal chance of surviving in what is often an unequal and unfair world.

How many times has deafness in a young child not been discovered until after observing that sharp or unexpected noises have been ignored? Despite the developments in clinical testing for hearing loss at an early age this still happens.

Think of the kind of noise that is usually made when a metal object, such as a knife, fork or a spoon, or even all three, are dropped on to a hard surface. To a profoundly deaf child no sound will have been heard at all. A severely deaf child may hear some degree of sound but not enough to warrant any immediate reaction. However, if either of them had been watching when this happened they may notice a pained expression on the face of the person who did hear the clatter!

The lesson learnt from this is that the action of dropping things can be unpleasant. Of course, it can be the wrong sort of lesson should the child try copying the action!

An alternative way for the child to learn how to 'hear' noise, and therefore understand it, is to give him an object, like the spoon, and guide him through the action of banging it against a hard surface. By placing his other hand on the surface - but well away from the intended point of impact - his touch will pick up the vibrations made when the spoon hits the surface. For reasons that should be obvious that kind of lesson is not recommended for the parent who longs for a quiet life!

All musical instruments vibrate and the range of vibrations produced can be felt as they are being played. The piano and the xylophone are particularly good examples. Likewise it is possible to discover the range of the human voice through this same sense of touch. Try resting the finger tips lightly against the throat next time you are speaking.

Through good family support and the kind of professional help referred to in earlier chapters all but the most severely multiple-disabled child can expect to receive a formal education as complete as any child with normal abilities.

Enlightened play-group leaders are trained to help children of mixed abilities and disabilities discover how to play and learn together. Modern technology can play an important part in this early learning process. Computer Play, for example, is designed to encourage reading skills and the uses of CD ROM.

Thanks to modern technology and enlightened teaching methods the majority of hearing-impaired and deaf children in full-time education will be able to go to mainstream primary and secondary schools. Some will need to attend Partially-Hearing Units that are special classrooms attached to mainstream schools. Qualified teachers of the deaf who are able to offer extra help with developing language as well as school subjects run these. For others, such as the profoundly deaf and the deafblind who need much more specialised help, there are special schools which have specialist teachers and other professional help available, such as from communicators and speech therapists.

Through this system a deaf child can achieve a good standard of education together with the added bonus of having received guidance in how to integrate with those who have full hearing. It is a far cry from the limited help that was available to earlier generations of deaf children and is to be commended for the way it has enabled today's young deaf people to have a greater quality of adult life. Nevertheless there is still much room for improvement.

For those who have spent from 10 to 12 years cocooned in a special education environment it can come as a great shock when they have to leave the school system behind them and venture out into an unfamiliar working world. It will be like having a constant and reliable prop suddenly removed from their side. Without help from such props they can almost literally fall down. The next two chapters should give some idea of how they can cope with and adapt to this change.

Further education is open to all who are academically able to follow this path but the level of communication support they will require may be far less than what they had become used to during their formative school years. The advent of the use of CD-ROMs and the range of other technical equipment now available has brought about welcome changes in the learning environment but there will always be a need for interpreters, lip-speakers and notetakers. These, combined with a sense of dedication and perseverance by the student, will bring about the desired result: that long-cherished qualification and gateway to a chosen career.

Not all classrooms or halls used for Adult Education classes are fitted out with loop or infrared systems nor are qualified interpreters readily available. It may, though, be possible to enlist some form of additional help through contact with representatives of a local group for the deaf or hearing-impaired. Those same people are able to give advice on the best form of personal sound-assistive equipment if this is preferred. The pleasure gained from learning new skills and from making new friends far outweighs any problems that may be experienced through communication difficulties.

Training Courses and Seminars can be coped with in a similar manner. The main difference to bear in mind is having to make allowances for seating and lighting arrangements. Seating that is incorrectly positioned can hamper not only comfort, and therefore concentration, but obscure hand movements by the interpreter if one is present. A well-lit meeting room makes lip-reading, sign language or reading of print far easier to follow but a room set up for presenting slides or video-type displays does not. Just try looking at both the screen presentation and at the speaker's face in a darkened room in order to follow every detail - an almost futile attempt! In a case like that a good loop system will be very helpful so long as it is not one that also picks up the dominating noise of the projector, the air conditioning system, or whatever.

For many people being able to drive a car has become an essential part of modern life and the ability of a deaf person wishing to do this should be no different from anyone else who is lawfully permitted to do so. The only problem they may have is in convincing an instructor that they are capable of coping with Car Driving Lessons, but that surely also applies to anyone with normal hearing? An inability to hear, or hear correctly, the instructions being given during the lesson is no different from any other learner driver's inability to listen.

A deaf learner driver has more fun than a hearing one. He can request instructions in mime or other recognisable visual descriptions, or handwritten or printed notes before taking the car out on to the road. And, if the instructor values his life well enough, it is a simple matter to indicate with hand movements, rather than speaking or shouting further instructions. Admittedly the instructor may sometimes find it rather difficult to stay calm enough in an emergency situation to remember the right signals!

As for developing those driving skills, the learner will quickly discover that he can feel the vibrations from the car engine when his feet rest on the foot controls. Through this experience he will often be ready to change gears before the long-suffering instructor has finished working out which signing method to use to explain the instruction. Another advantage a deaf driver has is the extra-visual skill he has developed as a result of his disability. This is so useful in anticipating the changes of driving conditions that occur during any car journey. Unfortunately this superior knowledge is not always appreciated by instructors and is best used as tactfully as possible.

By the time the learner driver is competent enough to take his driving test he will have acquired enough confidence from teaching his instructor the art of plain communication to be able to use this skill in advising and reassuring the unsuspecting examiner. Well, why not try it and see?

Advice on learning other skills, such as physical training, yoga and other health classes, dancing and sports, can be found in later chapters. It is possible that by reading on you can learn how to live life more to the full, although not necessarily be any the wiser.

CHAPTER SIX

GETTING A JOB

Long gone are the days when a deaf school-leaver or a newly deafened adult was expected to be employed in work that required little or no daily communication. Earlier chapters of this book will have shown how it is possible for them to cope with almost any type of work. There are still a few exceptions but at the present rate of progress in technical developments, together with determination on the part of the individual, even these restrictions will eventually be overcome.

Possibly the only real problem that a deaf or deafened person has to deal with after deciding which job to go after is finding the confidence to apply for the post which first caught their interest. This might not be too daunting for the more extrovert type but most of us need encouragement when it comes to persevering with applying for the kind of job we want to do. It is all too easy to give up after the first application has been turned down and, as is often the case, without any clear explanation.

There are all sorts of reasons for this lack of success and being deaf is unlikely to be at the top of the list. So what does go wrong?

Perhaps he or she failed to read or complete the application form properly, or he had the wrong kind of qualifications or experience. Was his handwriting legible? Would he have been available for the interview date specified? Or maybe it was simply that the employer disapproved of his hobby of playing in a pop group in his spare time? The list is almost endless but each one of these reasons could just as easily apply to someone with normal hearing. Most of these could have been avoided had the job application form been given serious attention in the first place.

These days, in theory at least, legislation exists to encourage employers to give as much consideration over job applications from deaf or otherwise disabled people as from those submitted by able-bodied ones. The same rules urge them to provide adequate facilities to help all employees do their jobs to the best of their ability. Many employers do follow such official guidelines but there will always be some who take the view that deafness or any other disability is a barrier to useful employment.

For this reason alone it is worthwhile applying to the government-run Employment Service for registration as a disabled person. Not only does registering help to open doors with prospective employers but all kinds of other help, including financial assistance where applicable, become more easily available. The Employment Service has Counselling Teams whose staff are able to advise both the applicant and the employer on the most appropriate kind of help. Many of the charities and organisations named in the Helplist are able to assist with making local contact.

Having read this far, you may feel confident enough to apply for that job. All you need to do now is to wait for the application form to arrive, fill it in and post it off. A piece of cake!

Or is it?

Of course it is. There is nothing to it. Just fill in the usual details: name, address, and qualifications - that sort of thing. Easy.

Well, it is if that is all the prospective employer is looking for. Unfortunately these days they like to have every little detail explained to them, which is why those forms are so often several pages in length. Even writing down your address can cause problems if you live some distance from the place of work, unless you can give reassurance that you will have no travel problems. Few people can honestly guarantee that, not even those living only a short distance away.

What about those qualifications you listed? On their own that information is rather basic but if there is room to write down why you chose those subjects or courses then this will help give the employer a far better insight into what you are like. Even writing about the ones in which you did not gain a qualification will show that you are willing to apply yourself to hard work. What is more you, yourself, will feel so much better for writing all these things down. The list will show exactly what you have achieved - all part of the confidence building process.

This confidence can take a sharp dive if you are applying for your first job and the next section on the form asks you for details of your previous employment. For the more imaginative individual, this should present no problem. Simply write down what you think you would do in an imaginary work situation and use the knowledge and information acquired from all that studying.

Poor imagination?

Then what about that time you helped out at Auntie Donna's snack bar last summer, or when you did a spell of shelf stacking at the local store? The jobs may bear no relation to the kind of work you are applying for but it is all useful and helpful information for the employer. Reading through what you have written down should put a stop to that ebbing confidence.

A word of caution though. All this is best drafted out first on a separate sheet of paper just in case you are unhappy with your first efforts. And the next - and the one after that. The last thing you want to do is to spoil an application form with the 'wrong kind of writing' - illegible scribble and covered with crossings out.

A great deal of the advice given so far on completing job application forms applies to anyone, with or without hearing. There is just one slight problem that may specifically apply to applicants with poor hearing, but not necessarily so. Extra care must be taken to use correct grammar and spelling when writing things down.

You do? Are you sure?

Just stop and think about the difference between the spoken and written words. How many people actually say '*I have*'? They may put that down on paper but what is usually said is '*I've*'. Another example is '*I am going*': the spoken version is '*I'm going*'. Similarly, '*I have got*'' is spoken as '*I've got*'.

But what does all this have to do with filling in job application forms?

It can make a big difference when you realise that people with a below normal level of hearing will seldom catch the sounds at the ends of words. If they are not corrected each time then they may well go through life thinking that it is normal to speak or write '*I got*' or '*I go*'. This may give the impression that they have had a very limited education when the opposite is probably true.

What to do about it?

Get practising, of course. And what better way to do it than to pop along to the local library and browse through a selection of books off the fiction shelves. No matter if it is a Mills & Boon, a gothic horror, or something written by authors like Micky Spillane, Ruth Rendell or John le Carré. Just read through them, learn how the words are used and possibly even enjoy the stories as well.

The day will come when that much awaited letter arrives inviting you to attend for an interview. What next?

Well, after you have finished dancing up and down the hall and the dog has stopped chasing its tail round and round in excitement it will be time to think ahead about the next stage - what to wear.

These days most employers attach less importance to this aspect of the interview but a good first impression still counts. A building site employer may not be too impressed if you turn up wearing your best suit but nor is he likely to think much of those gaping fashion holes in the jeans you chose to put on instead. It could give him the wrong idea of your standard of workmanship. If, on the other hand, the interview is for a post in an office where business of a serious nature is conducted then it is not advisable to turn up in your brightest coloured clothes nor in the minimal size range and with your face adorned with a distracting assortment of jewellery. Save them for the celebration party after you have been offered the job.

For the interview itself you really need a crash course in how to act. It is certainly one way to succeed in hiding your nervousness. But then why should you be nervous? You have done your homework for this job and, thanks to all that practice in completing and presenting the application form in the right kind of way, you have confidence in your ability to see things through. This will show just by the way you walk through that door.

You will be smiling your greeting instead of grimacing, or at least you should be. You will be ready to shake hands instead of trembling; and to take the seat offered to you with gracious acceptance instead of flopping down in nervous exhaustion. In fact you will give such a good impression of paying attention to everything that is being said to you that you may even get away with the interviewer not realising you are deaf.

One young lady received a great deal of praise over her attentive attitude when being interviewed for a temporary post. The employer never did discover the real reason why she had sat on the edge of her seat. Not only could she hardly hear what he was saying, but she had found him difficult to lip-read! Yes, she got the job.

It is all about confidence. Take each situation one step at a time. Never be afraid to ask the interviewer/employer to repeat what he or she has said. It will sound a perfectly natural question especially if the interview is being conducted in a room where there is an unavoidable amount of background noise or other distractions. Remember that the employer may be finding this equally disruptive. There is nothing worse than pretending to have understood what was said and ending up talking at cross-purposes.

If it is necessary to mention in advance about having hearing difficulties or circumstances make the situation obvious, such as needing to have an Interpreter in attendance or your Hearing Dog with you, then do so but try to keep the explanations as short as possible. Leave the questions to the interviewer. He, or she, will learn a great deal more about you by the way you answer and discuss any possible problems and the situation is likely to make the interview far more interesting. Remember that you are the expert on what you can and cannot cope with and by having that knowledge you will impress with your confidence.

All this does not necessarily mean you will get that first job just like that - but when you do you should find the information in the following chapter very helpful.

CHAPTER SEVEN

THE WORK ENVIRONMENT

Why do we go out to work?

What a silly question! To earn enough money to live on, of course - well, most of us do!

Then what about those who already have enough income from other sources but still go out to work in an unpaid capacity. Why do they bother?

For some, voluntary work is the only chance they have to mix with people outside the comfort and security of their homes. They also do it because they enjoy the work.

So, what about the idea of enjoying going out to work and being paid for it? If you have acted on some of the suggestions made in the last chapter you will be halfway to doing just that.

Only halfway? That is because the rest is down to you and all that confidence you worked at so hard to build.

You are the only one who knows what kind of support and help you need. Few employers or colleagues are mind readers and so it is down to you to communicate and ask.

Noise is an unavoidable part of everyday life for most people. This may present few problems for those profoundly deaf but the severely deaf are more likely to pick up some sort of background noise rather than human speech - machinery, generators, music, building work - both outside and inside their place of work.

At work there are laws - called the Noise at Work Regulations - that aim to protect your hearing. All employers are bound by them to have noise levels assessed and to keep a record of the assessment. By law they must make every effort to reduce noise levels as far as possible and provide ear protectors where necessary. If working in excessively noisy conditions is a part of the daily work then the employer must arrange for your hearing to be tested regularly by experts. It is just the same for those who spend long hours in front of VDUs (Visual Display Units) - they need to have regular checks on their eyesight.

Special attention has to paid to those working in hazardous areas. It has not always been possible to allow a deaf person to work in such places because of the likelihood of their failure to hear warnings.

There are certain noises that for safety reasons must be heard, such as alarm signals or bells in cases of emergencies. Modern technology has produced flashing lights and vibrator alarms, such as the Deaf Alerter system. The pagers provided with the latter can also be programmed to act as personal pagers. These can be part financed through the Employment Agency although not all employers are able or willing to commit themselves to these extra facilities, particularly the owners of small businesses.

Working in shops and stores with the sound of the electronic cash tills beeping away can be very stressful to the hearing-aid user. This is an employment area with some way to go in considering all aspects of the needs of disabled people.

Communication at work can be either fraught with difficulties or enormous fun, depending on how you choose to approach the problem. Only those trained to speak clearly at all times, such as actors, programme presenters, teachers, will know to how to make themselves understood at all times. After all in their line of business every word counts.

There seem to be far too many people who do not know how, or cannot be bothered, to speak clearly. Those whose living it is to answer telephones do try to make the effort but more often than not this is because it is natural for them to do so and not as a result of good training. In the workplace a deaf person can often get by with lip reading but not always, especially when colleagues or workmates are not aware of the rule to face you when speaking. It can be quite fun though trying to dance around him or her to get into the ideal face to face position for lip-reading. Eye contact is one of the key tools for effective communication.

There may well be occasions when that form of communication just does not work and the ideal alternative is an offer to write things down. A helpful colleague's ability to adapt to using both face to face communication and writing down notes, or even using a form of mime or sign language when necessary, is much appreciated and should be encouraged. Conducted in the right surroundings it is a natural way to make contact without causing social embarrassment or loss of dignity. It can also be great entertainment and lighten up an otherwise dull working day.

Background noise can be a terrible distraction whatever the work situation and trying to use a telephone in those conditions is no exception. Telephone receivers are not designed to reduce or eliminate such noises in the way that a normal functioning human ear can do and so ways and means have to be found to avoid this difficulty as far as possible. Although it is not always practical to reduce or shut off background noise before responding to telephone calls a lot can be done by both the caller and the person receiving the call to ensure that the voice is channelled directly into the mouthpiece. It may not always be possible or practical to sit or stand up straight when answering a call but the practice of cradling the receiver between the ear and the shoulder is no help at all. It strangles the voice sounds, making clear speech impossible.

Neither is it a good idea for the receiver to be held well away from the face when speaking, the mouthpiece will then also pick up background noise and too little of the voice of the speaker. Shouting is useless since the louder the voice is raised the more distorted the speech becomes. The caller may then resort to what can only be described as childspeak that would be utterly demoralising for the listener. If everyone was to think about how they physically used the telephone when speaking it would put into perspective the right approach to make when communicating face to face.

Taking unfamiliar telephoned messages for colleagues can be difficult to make sense of at the best of times, especially if you know little or nothing about the subject and/or the caller is one of those speakers in urgent need of training in how to use a telephone. Taking calls for your own work range is usually easier since you are likely to be familiar enough with the subject to pick out those key words that help you to conduct a reasonably intelligent line of conversation.

Sympathetic colleagues are usually happy to help out with difficult phone calls but how much more satisfying it would be to handle all calls yourself if you were to have access to a specially adapted telephone? Not all employers can afford to provide these but laws now in force are designed to ensure that equal opportunities are available to all disabled employees.

There are many different types of technical aids available, at cost, and most have been described in Chapter 4. Computer technology has pushed the old barriers wide open so that even profoundly deaf people can communicate easily and quickly with the hearing world at the touch of a few buttons. The use of the E-mail and Internet systems have become so popular that even people with normal hearing prefer to use it as an easier alternative to the telephone. In time it may well overtake the use of fax machines which have served so well to transmit both hand-written and typed messages.

For any business, large or small, to remain successful it is essential that employees are given the necessary training to do their jobs properly. Large companies are able to arrange their own in-house training programmes, but smaller businesses depend a great deal on support and help from outside courses held elsewhere. Whichever option is followed this kind of help is given in many forms and is, or should be, available to all employees whether classed as disabled or not.

Portable loop systems, as previously described, are available to pick up speech at conferences, lectures, training courses, etc. Modern hearing-aids have been improved so that when used in conjunction with loop systems there is less interference from picking up irritating background noises - unless the person sitting next to the system's microphone is in the habit of constantly tapping a pencil or drumming his fingers on something hard.

The disadvantage of some types of portable loop systems is the need to lay out the lengthy cabling around the perimeter of the meeting or lecture room prior to the start of the meeting or lecture. It can also create a safety hazard if the loop cable is not stuck securely down to the floor with masking tape before someone has a very good trip. Also, the positioning of the microphone and control box depends upon the distance to the nearest power point since the supply cable used can only be stretched so far without causing a safety hazard. Some designs incorporate the volume control into the control box, which is fine if you are sitting close by. If you are several seats away from it and you urgently need to adjust the volume control then you could have a distressing problem. Pre-arranged sign language with the person sitting nearest to the control box is helpful but even the best laid plans can go wrong!

A Conference Folder of the type suitable for use in medium-size meetings rooms would eliminate most of the problems encountered with using a loop system that depends on great lengths of cable but can be expensive to buy.

Lectures, talks or demonstrations which use slides or video projections can be difficult to follow without some form of subtitling or projected text to outline the main points being described. The use of projectors means that rooms have to be darkened in order to see what is on the screen. This makes it almost impossible to lip-read the speaker or lecturer and because the operation noise from the projector is picked up by some loop systems it can dominate any commentary spoken softly.

Group staff training can be conducted by making the best use of seating arrangements to aid visual understanding of what is being said. Visual can mean lip-reading, use of flip-charts and paper copy handouts, or all three.

One to one training can and should be offered especially where computer training is involved. It is just not possible to lip-read the demonstrator and look at the keyboard or personal monitor at the same time.

Training is a learning process that can work both ways. By observing how you try to cope with the additional problems which deafness can bring to a job colleagues and employers can learn the extent of the problems. This may encourage them to think of further and perhaps better solutions and so help to increase your confidence. Confident workers are happy ones, able to create a good working environment for all. No bad way to improve business!

Colleagues should be able to make the deaf person aware of their being spoken to by giving a light tap on the arm or shoulder. It is important to do this correctly since it is all too easy for an unexpected touch to cause sheer fright - the equivalent of creeping up behind an hearing person and then shouting out *'Boo!'* Another problem is how to avoid having the action misconstrued since there is an alarming modern trend to regard such physical contact as a matter for litigation in the courts. As colleagues and fellow workers learn how to lip-speak they will, and without being aware of it, do so clearly and face the person they are speaking to without the need to be reminded - an advantage all round.

Deafness should not be a barrier to making a career change. Technology is rapidly changing everything and thus making more choices of work accessible. Society's attitude, especially amongst the older generation, towards deafness and disability in general is taking longer to change and therefore to learn how to help but in many areas employers are encouraged to link with local community projects which organise sign language and lip-reading courses, and Deaf Awareness training.

Thanks to the widespread involvement of schools that accommodate special needs educational units younger people receive Deaf Awareness training to help them to be more adaptable. They can also receive a certain amount of financial help through the Employment Service, in conjunction with the employer, to obtain the additional technical aids they may need for their career or job training.

For employers to comprehend the real needs of the deaf or deafened this can only be resolved by example from more outgoing members of the deaf community.

CHAPTER EIGHT

THE HOME ENVIRONMENT

A man's house is his castle... he can pull up the drawbridge and relax behind the safety of solid, well-fortressed walls. Well, that is what the lawyer Sir Edward Coke argued in 1628, but that was in the days before door-to-door salesmen had the country gripped by the throat and no-one had yet thought up the idea of telephones.

What was more, he could leave the mundane but hazardous tasks such as cooking and laundering to the lady of the house - sorry, castle - or even to servants, whether paid or otherwise. Visitors, when they were allowed across the draw-bridge, were entertained by hired musicians, dances, or games - none of this electronically produced powerhouse form of entertainment which bombards the ears of those living in the highly civilised twenty-first century. Poor Modern Man - or Woman! How would he or she cope without all the gadgetry that depends upon the use of electricity in order to function? Not very well, in fact.

Unexpected, and possibly uninvited, door-callers have a habit of arriving just as something is about to boil over in the kitchen, or an interesting programme on the television or radio is about to start. This is not too much of a problem for a hearing person, as it is a simple matter of moving from one area of the house to another with minimum disruption to the routine in order to answer the door. For the deaf person this can be a major undertaking.

For a start, he or she may be unaware that the saucepan is about to boil over unless he is already watching it or can smell the increase in temperature as the contents rise up to the top of the pan. The doorbell could go unheard, of course, in which case there would be no cause for getting in a flap - unless someone else also in the house had ignored it on the assumption that the other was going to open the door. Not too much of a problem if the caller had been that unwanted salesman but what if it had been Cousin Edward dropping by on the off-chance while he was in the neighbourhood? Oh, the arguments that would follow - well, you know what families can be like!

As for the deaf person settling down to follow a television programme just as the doorbell goes, he is likely to either strangle himself with his neck loop if he is using one and tries to get up in a hurry or break the headphones for his infra-red sound system when he throws them down in haste. Without doubt such aids are a marvellous way of following televised or sound broadcasts, or for listening to music played on the home entertainment unit - but door-callers and telephone-callers rarely wait long enough for the deaf person to disentangle himself to get to the door or phone in time. Door and telephone bells can be fitted with flashing lights but they can still make you jump when they start up, just as any sudden loud noises do.

The specially adapted telephones mentioned in earlier chapters are truly a great help but just as with ordinary phones they do not prepare you for the unfamiliar voices of strangers. The harsh rapid speech of telephone sales callers are a particular cross to bear. However, it may be reassuring to learn that those with poor hearing do have one big advantage when it comes to dealing with unwanted callers. By the time they have asked the caller to repeat their message between six to eight times in order to understand what they are trying to sell it is generally the salesperson who ends up slamming down the receiver in exasperation.

As anyone with normal hearing will tell you the kitchen area is notorious for the amount of harsh clattering sounds produced. The clink and clatter of crockery and cutlery on hard surfaces and the clanging of metal saucepans can be almost too painful to bear. Worse if something is dropped or smashed - not only does the noise have to be coped with but the upset created by the damage or breakage as well.

A hearing-aid wearer can always turn this off and work in peaceful bliss but family or other visitors to the kitchen may find this a selfish attitude, especially when they want to make themselves understood above the din. Of course, if they complain too much they run the risk of being told to do the job themselves. Which is probably why those irksome boring jobs like vacuum-cleaning literally shatter the household peace. You just cannot win when a deaf person is around.

For reasons of hygiene most kitchens have hard surfaces - it makes them easier to clean. As a consequence noises sound harsher and voices may echo, making it almost impossible for the deaf person to hold an intelligent conversation with those nearest. If they depend upon lip-reading to complement what they can hear then they are in danger of cutting, bruising, or scalding themselves as they try to do this at the same time as getting on with the task in hand. Since not everyone can or wants to use a dish-washing machine trying to hold a conversation while washing the dishes has its own set of problems. The 'you wash and I'll dry' rule seldom works since it is difficult for most people to hear speech clearly over the clatter of cutlery and crockery from the draining-board and the sink. It is also extremely difficult to aim for the draining-board if the person washing-up is constantly turning round to follow what a speaker is saying - not everyone can afford to replace the dinner-service every month.

Carpets or carpet tiles on the floors of most living-rooms and comfortable well-placed seating arrangements will not only make visitors feel more welcome but are the best way to reduce the harshness of sounds. Likewise will curtains and any other soft furnishings made of heavy, rather than lightweight, materials. Colour schemes should be kept as light as possible since the more light in a room the better it will be to see people's faces for lip-reading. They will also make it easier to avoid walking into the pet dog or cat spread-eagled across the floor. Just how light or bright depends upon your level of enthusiasm for regular interior redecorating.

Floorcoverings in kitchens should be suitable for easy mopping up jobs since washing-machines and dishwashers have a nasty habit of breaking down and sinks become blocked up and overflow. The same advice applies to those who live in areas where flooding may occur after heavy rainfalls. Tiled floors are easy to mop dry but a well-cushioned washable vinyl one is better at helping to cut down the noise level. It will also soften the fall of cutlery and crockery and reduce the amount of breakages. Not everyone agrees with the idea of curtains being put up at the kitchen window but they are another good way of reducing the level of background noise.

The one common agony to be endured by deaf and hearing alike is the widespread use of powered tools. You name it and it is being used by someone, somewhere and at almost any time of the day or night - DIY, private building construction, home and street cleaning, garden maintenance - the list is endless. A profoundly deaf person will experience no more than the vibrations of the tool or machinery in use, and a hearing-aid user can switch off - a situation than can cause danger to themselves or to others if they are not visually aware of what is happening.

To the uninitiated ironing can be a very boring job. It is the main reason why many with normal hearing will resort to switching on the kitchen radio or television for something to listen to while they work. A person with enough hearing to cope can listen to either of these by using headphones or a neck loop connected to the sound system. They do, though, run a serious risk of strangling, burning, or electrocuting themselves if the lead to the electric iron becomes entangled with any additional cables they may need to use to listen to the programme. The alternative is to either persuade someone else to do the job or give up ironing altogether. Few modern garments need ironing anyway.

Not everyone can live with a pet animal in the house - and sometimes the feeling is mutual. Hearing Dogs for the deaf are a wonderful way for a dog lover to have independence since these animals are trained to act as a four-legged pair of extra ears. They are not quite skilled enough at opening doors to complete strangers but they will let their owners know when there is a visitor waiting at the front door or the telephone is ringing. They will also act as alarm clocks, useful for those who have to get up in time to go to work or have a particular train to catch. With a Hearing Dog around the home many kitchen accidents can be avoided for they will understand when a saucepan or kettle is about to boil over, and give warning. Since no dog, or any other pet, is perfect it is important to remember to keep out of their reach anything that is easily chewable or removed. Hearing aids left laying around have been known to come to a sorry and expensive end.

Cats are another matter. As well as being almost untrainable they are also unreliable - a sad state of affairs for cat lovers. They are only good as alarm clocks when they want to be fed or let out of the home to attend the calls of nature. They will sit on, or pat or poke hard at, their owner's face several minutes before the early morning alarm clock is due to vibrate or flash. The same cat will stay curled up and sound asleep when a doorbell or telephone rings.

A deaf person cannot hear if the water header tank is filling up. If the tank is left to empty unchecked then this can lead to the hot water tank being allowed to burn dry. It is a good idea to make regular checks on the level of the water pressure in use and not leave it to 'wait and see'.

For the first-time hearing-aid user the once familiar home can change literally at the flick of a switch and making it feel menacing. With so many new sounds and noises to be heard it is helpful to have someone around with whom they can discuss what they hear. Sometimes hearing-aids pick up noises from sources which are not at first obvious, especially when the wearer is experimenting with the level of volume control. Humming noises may be picked up from all manner of electrical gadgets, and not just in their own home but from the neighbours as well. Even voices from other people's mobile phones and personal stereos may be clearly heard. Reassurance is needed that these noises in the head are not tinnitus taking over completely, or the first signs of madness, or both.

For those who are deafblind there are many gadgets or tools that help them to maintain their independence and their sanity. There are pens for putting raised bumps on virtually any surface - tea and coffee jars, cooker controls or light switches. A liquid-level indicator bleeps when the container is filled to the right level and so helps to avoid spills in the kitchen. Plastic guards help to guide fingers when that ironing task can be put off no longer.

For those with residual hearing there are talking clocks or watches, televisions without a screen for listening only, and (very important!) a warning device that buzzes when it starts to rain - useful for getting in the nearly dry washing before it gets wet through again!

Perhaps a man's home is his castle after all - a place where he may feel protected and secure.

CHAPTER NINE

SHOPPING AND BUSINESS TRIPS

A great many problems are encountered by the deaf when out shopping or attending to business affairs which could be avoided if there was more co-operation and understanding from the hearing members of retail and business organisations.

Few stores or shops are customer friendly for those who have a daily struggle in coping with a normal hearing world. There are well-intentioned training programmes arranged by some of the larger organisations and some staff in many of the smaller shops make a personal effort to help, but it is not enough. As a consequence many deaf shoppers will do little more than make a quick visit to the nearest self-service store where they can purchase basic goods and keep conversation with sales assistants to a minimum.

Unfriendly? Of course, but for them it is the least traumatic way to shop and still preserve their sanity. Were all shops and stores to train their staff in fully understanding the problems of deafness then, with the number of deaf people estimated at more than eight million in the United Kingdom alone, surely their sales figures would rocket skywards?

From a shop assistant's point of view it can be difficult to tell whether a person is deaf or simply giving a display of bad manners. The only way the assistant may realise is when she or he attempts to speak to the customer.

To an outsider a deaf person will seem to be the most relaxed of shoppers since as they may not hear what is going on around them, or very little, they are not easily distracted from the purpose of their shopping trip - but more of that later.

Often it is the hearing-aid user who endures, and can cause, the most stress in a shopping environment. In theory they can be recognised by the hearing-aid, or aids, they wear but in practice may not always be so easy to spot. Not only that but many older users, especially those who have become deaf and introduced to hearing-aids late in life, hate being seen wearing an aid and may leave it at home. Even if a hearing-aid is noticed it may not necessarily be working. Sometimes the user forgets to switch it on or put a battery in it. If the old battery has run down they may have left the spare one at home.

For the hearing-aid user the most carefully planned shopping or business trip can turn into a nightmare. The journey to the shops will have brought its own problems, especially if some distance has to be travelled. Car journeys, particularly if the shopper is doing the driving, need extra concentration and the car park attendant at the car park may not be the best of communicators. Bus journeys, whilst needing far less concentration during the travel stage, still have the problem of comprehending the speech of bored, tired drivers to overcome -

public service operators seem to have missed out on deaf awareness training. One way of avoiding a difficult conversation with the bus driver is to have exactly the right bus fare to hand. This practice can backfire if the fares have gone up yet again.

Once in the town, or shopping area, the volume control on the hearing-aid has to be quickly turned down, or even switched off, before the high level of traffic noise threatens to destroy what hearing is left. One of the worst but unintentional offenders are vehicles used by the different emergency services. Their warning sirens, which are so essential, blare out with a shrillness and harshness that can bring tears of pain to the eyes of a hearing-aid user and a short sharp visual shock to those blissfully unaware of any noise. People with normal hearing can suffer too but their ability to select and interpret the difference in sounds lessens the shock to their nervous system.

Even in the pedestrianised shopping areas there are the unexpected hazards of maintenance and late delivery vehicles which slowly crawl along almost unseen until they are at your side. True they will have made little noise, making a hearing-aid wearer believe that his aid has stopped functioning, but the suddenness of their appearance can make him jump three feet into the air.

Unexpected traffic in these so-called safe areas are not the only problems to watch out for. The trend for street sales canvassing can be particularly distracting and tiring as well as time-consuming when there may be little time to spare. Complete strangers approach with clipboard or leaflets in hand but with so much background noise and constant distracting crowd movements it can be almost impossible to work out the speech sounds being made. In situations like this lip-reading can be a disadvantage as the eye contact so necessary for it can be mistaken for an expression of genuine interest in what is being sold or offered. The completely deaf have a similar problem, as they will be trying to read any material being displayed.

Many local authorities have gone some way to making it safer for pedestrians and cyclists to cross busy roads but there can still be problems. All members of the public can cross safely at traffic lights and pedestrian crossings when a green light comes on, in the shape of a 'green man'. The same system will also emit a series of warning beeps for the benefit of pedestrians who have poor eyesight or are blind and the waiting areas have textured paving for the feet to sense easily. This is not always appreciated by those wearing thin-soled or flimsy shoes or who have painfully arthritic toe joints.

Seeking quiet sanctuary in a shop where the hearing aid volume can be returned to its more normal level is not always possible. Few shops or stores seem to be without some kind of nerve-jangling 'mood' music being played in the background. You do not have to be old to have a difference of opinion on what is 'mood' music.

Completely deaf shoppers do not have this problem but their eye and neck muscles will ache from constant watching out for unexpected traffic and people hazards along the High Street. Many hearing aid wearers experience similar physical stresses, especially by those who are under a constant strain to lip-read in their attempt to sort out every noise they hear into words and speech. Shop or store assistants who dare to complain aloud of similar aches and pains do so at their peril.

There is nothing a deaf - or deafened - person hates more than to be shouted at or simple requests to be spoken to more clearly and slowly met with blank stares. The way some less enlightened shop and other business staff react can make the customer want to flee the shop before the men in white coats are called in to take them away.

The policy of playing background music in stores and shops may well be considered a relaxing way of encouraging shoppers to part with more money - but relaxing for whom? To a hearing-aid user it sounds more like a terrible racket of incomprehensible noise. What with that and the constant dominating beeps from the electronic cash registers it is almost impossible to hear a shop assistant's reply when enquiring about the goods on offer. Even if the customer does catch some of what was said there is no guarantee that he or she understood, especially if the assistant was looking down or away during much of the conversation. The resulting misunderstanding can mean red faces, bad feeling and possible loss of custom.

Poor acoustics is another obstacle. In stores and shops which stock packaged goods, such as self-service premises that sell groceries or toiletries, the noise is likely to be doubled by the echoes that bounce back off almost every hard surface. In contrast soft materials on display such as fashion clothes or soft furnishings create much quieter surroundings and are therefore more pleasant to visit. The biggest drawback can be the tendency to not only use subdued lighting but to invite almost too much comfort. Who has never succumbed to the testing of comfortable armchairs, sofas or even beds on display in showrooms?

Poorly thought out shop lighting is a hazard not just for people with poor eyesight. If it is shop or store policy to have good lighting positioned over the sale goods on offer then why not over every sales counter or desk as well? It is almost impossible to lip-read in dimly lit rooms or clearly see the faces of sales staff. Reading faces is second nature to many deaf people and those staff who somehow manage to maintain eye contact with a customer whilst also trying to package or wrap goods and handle the payment transaction are worth their weight in gold. Their help is equally welcome when trying to find out how much to pay when the till screen is not easily in view and so avoid embarrassing misunderstandings. Better still if there is a well-trained and patient assistant willing to write things down.

There is in existence a Sympathetic Hearing Scheme, represented in many public-use places by an 'ear' graphic. Its aim is to inform the deaf customer that trained staff and help facilities are available to give a hearing-help service. Unfortunately this arrangement is not as successful as it could be. Not all deaf people, or staff, are aware of its existence or how best to use it. Staff trained to help move on or leave and in the cut and thrust of modern businesses few employers find the time to ensure continuity in awareness of the Scheme.

Banks and building societies and some post offices, with their head-high Perspex safety screens, can be notorious for displaying the ear graphic over a counter that is closed - often the only one specially wired up to a loop system. No wonder some shoppers enter stores and shops in a bad mood after spending a frustrating amount of time trying to understand what the bank clerk was saying at the 'normal use' counter. People in wheelchairs, especially those out and about independently in battery-operated ones, have an even more difficult time trying to conduct their business. Most counters are too high for them to reach properly and if their hearing is poor it can be extremely difficult for them to make that all-important eye contact essential to good lip-reading.

With any business premises that display the Scheme's ear symbol, including shops and stores, it is only natural for a customer to assume that the staff, or at least some of them, will have been instructed in deaf awareness training. What a let down this can be when the first sales assistant approached has never heard of the Scheme and worse, thinks it all one huge joke.

How wonderful it would be for deaf people to know that they could set out on a shopping trip knowing that they would be able to enjoy it, be free to walk into any shop or store without dread, be treated on equal terms and made to feel like a normal human being.

CHAPTER TEN

BEING A PART OF THE COMMUNITY

There was a time when deaf people were kept in the background and ignored, placed on the same intelligence level as small children or classed with those regarded as mentally deficient or disadvantaged. As a consequence for many years the only way they could be involved in working with or helping the rest of the community was with their own kind - that is, the deaf with the deaf.

This situation is changing, and for the better. It is all due to the hard work and influence of a number of people, including some in public prominence, many of whom themselves became deaf or deafened in adult life often when at the peak of highly successful careers.

The change in attitudes has been brought about in two ways. The personal example of well-known people, and some less so, from all walks of life demonstrating how deaf people can be a useful part of the community. A series of innovative legislation introduced by successive governments in recent years has often been the result of long hours of debate and arguments put forward by some of the more popular politicians on behalf of the disabled people they have championed.

These actions are proof in themselves that deaf people should be encouraged to participate in decision making of any kind. Legislation is making it necessary for reviews to be carried out on the special needs requirements for all disabled people in places of public access. Employers and administrators of public buildings are being encouraged to invite employees and representatives of the disabled community to sit in on Review Committees. These special needs advisers have much personal experience from which they are able to point out aspects of a problem not previously realised. They can teach people with normal abilities how to act on their behalf

Few people understand how to communicate effectively as part of a team and much time is wasted in endless debate at meetings. Each individual member will be set on expressing his or her own point of view and ignoring or failing to listen to others. In addition to that people become careless over the way they speak and vary the pitch of their voices according to their state of wakefulness or health. The pace of the debate can make it difficult for even those with normal hearing to follow the conduct and content of the meeting.

Deaf people are much better at communicating than many hearing people. They perform in this rôle so well that they may be mistaken for trained members of the acting profession. Follow their example and observe the apparent confidence they have in pointing out how a team can work together. Review committees or any other kind of meeting can produce positive results and inspirational conclusions. What is more a successful special needs adviser will become a much valued member of the team.

As mentioned in earlier chapters, advancements in digital technology have made an enormous difference to the lives of disabled people. Computer systems and telephone improvements have done much to break down the barriers of communication and the use of the various types of loop systems and interpreters enables many more of the deaf community to meet the hearing world on equal terms.

Being part of the community means not just taking an active part in meetings but participating as a member of a Court jury, going to the Polling Station to vote, and voluntary work such as hospital visiting or involvement with registered charities and other kinds of voluntary organisations. There are also many opportunities to pass on and teach skills to others.

People with hearing disabilities are not excused from Jury service for cases held in the Crown Court. There are options available for the assistance of deaf jurors in courts but the discretion to allow any type of available assistance, or any person to sit as a juror, ultimately rests with the trial judge in each individual case. The Court Service does try to take into account possible problems for disabled jurors.

Jurors are summoned from all people whose names appear on the Electoral Roll who are aged between 18 and 70 years and have been living in the United Kingdom, the Channel Islands, or the Isle of Man for a period of at least five years since the age of 13. This means that it is more than likely that a deaf or hearing-impaired person will be called at some time or other. For that reason the Court concerns itself with making reasonable provisions for them.

Induction Loop systems are installed for the benefit hearing-aid users attending at the Crown Court. The Court Service liaison officer will endeavour to help in other ways, such as with the provision of Computer Aided Transcription. This is a system that allows a deaf person to have the court proceedings relayed to him or her simultaneously in written form.

Unfortunately sign language interpreters are no longer considered an option. The Lord Chief Justice has decided that it is not right for an independent person - for example, an interpreter - not sworn in as a member of the Jury, to retire with the jury. Although the interpreter would be there purely to relay what was being discussed he or she would be bound to take a part even though not expressing any personal opinion.

The provision of a signer would not be of benefit because the intonation of what is being said could not be conveyed. This is an essential aspect of preparing legal judgements.

When considering options for making arrangements to assist deaf jurors the needs of the individual must be taken into account. Every Crown Court has a Customer Service officer who should be contacted well in advance if information is needed on the facilities available or if help is required when visiting the court. The Court Service is committed to improving the quality of the service it provides and is always interested in the views and suggestions of court users in setting future standards.

Although microphones are set out in the Crown Court this is not always the case in the Magistrates Court. This is partly compensated by the different seating arrangements but it is still not always easy to hear what is going on.

The restructuring of the National Health Service has meant that the majority of patients have to stay in hospitals that may be many miles from their homes. Consequently their families and friends can find it too much of a strain, or too time-consuming, because of other family commitments to travel long distances for regular hospital visits. As a consequence people who are good listeners and communicators are always welcome as hospital visitors, helping to ease those long lonely and often stressful hours away from the familiar surroundings of home.

Deaf people, with their experience of the different ways of communication with young and old alike are particularly appreciated. All too often those hospital patients in most need of help are suffering from age-related hearing loss in addition to whatever medical condition brought about their hospital stay. They can be particularly lonely, as well as frightened, and few hospital staff however well-meaning have the time to develop the skill of speaking to them in a more normal adult way. So, what better visitor could they have than someone who will sit and talk with them without shouting or using childspeak, or are happy to write things down or use simple miming or sign language gestures. True, for those visitors who are hearing-aid users there is a certain amount of background noise to cope with, but a little perseverance will bring its own reward.

From hospital visiting to passing on and teaching skills to others is but a short step to helping others make more of their lives. Whatever practical skill is taught, the best results are achieved by one-to-one communication and personal example.

Craftwork, basket-work, woodwork, needle-craft, knitting, computer skills - these are only some of the things which deaf people can teach, and with more patience than most. And that is without mentioning other possibilities such as teaching lip-reading, signing or offering Deaf Awareness advice to businesses and the local community in general.

All upright and dutiful citizens will seize the opportunity to vote at General and Local elections. Won't they? Well, they may if they know which option is best suited for them to do so.

For some the event is treated like a social occasion, especially if the station is not far from the local pub: not for them the faceless option of postal or electronic voting.

A disadvantage of going out to a Polling Station to vote is the fact that the polling booths are often positioned inside dimly-lit halls or rooms that have poor acoustic quality. This can make it difficult to understand what the polling clerks are saying. The procedure these officers go through to check through the list of names they have that will identify you tends to be conducted with great solemness. The lack of facial expression can make would-be voters, deaf or hearing, feel that they are doing something wrong.

For those who take the family pet along with them to these places the reception given can be mixed. Guide Dogs for the Blind are more easily recognised and accepted but Hearing Dogs can take a lot more explaining. If the polling clerks are not dog lovers then there could be a problem - the adage that pets and children are a good way of breaking an icy atmosphere may be put severely to the test.

One lady went off to vote at her local Polling Station blissfully unaware that her pet Siamese cat, a creature renowned for its loud voice and friendly manner, was following her until she was most of the way there. Instead of turning round and taking it home, once she realised, she opted to pick it up and carry it the rest of the way. The reception at the Polling Station was mixed. Most were in favour of such enthusiasm and happy to fuss, except for one. It was all this particular polling clerk could do not back right away to safety or flee from the hall.

CHAPTER ELEVEN

COPING WITH HEALTH APPOINTMENTS

Most of us at some time in our lives will need to visit a doctor when we feel unwell or a dentist when something is wrong with our teeth. Some will make visits to practitioners of other medical treatments such as physiotherapy and homeopathy. Others, needing more specialist help, will attend hospital clinics.

Whichever it is we all have to go through the process of arranging appointments, sitting about in waiting rooms, talking with and listening to the practice staff and the practitioners, and coping with the treatment when this is necessary.

The first thing most of us do when we are feeling unwell is make an appointment to see the doctor. We can either call in at the medical practice or centre in person to do this or use the telephone. If we are too ill to do either, we may ask someone to arrange this on our behalf. These options apply to the deaf and hearing alike.

Calling in person to speak with the receptionist or the nurse is the best way to avoid misunderstandings when arranging an appointment. Most practices are busy and reception staff have to fit in the appointments process in between handling incoming phone calls, dealing with requests from other practice staff and seeing that patients are told when it is their turn to see the doctor or whoever.

All this activity creates a lot of background noise and distractions that can make communication difficult with anyone, whether their hearing is good or not. Trying to maintain eye contact for lip-reading can be difficult in this kind of situation.

Perseverance and patience is often the only answer but hard to find when you are feeling tired and unwell.

The alternative, of telephoning, is useful if the practice is some distance away or is out of the way from the usual route to the shops or to work. It does not eliminate the background noises coming from around the reception area. The receptionist or nurse can do little about that but at least there are no physical distractions to divert concentration. Well, not from the goings on at the practice end of the line but anything can be happening at the home end and usually does.

Asking someone else to make the appointment for you can bring its own problems. If it is that nice friendly neighbour from down the road, then half the day may pass by and two or three cups of tea or coffee consumed while she gives you sympathy and all the local gossip before the errand is done. You could feel a whole lot worse or better by that time.

If you rely on a textphone for making telephone calls then the BT Typetalk service can be of help. This was referred to in an earlier chapter.

Waiting-rooms are the best places for observing how the other half suffers, deciding what might be wrong with them, planning menus, thinking up new ideas for resolving problems or working out how to get revenge on the office manager. Well-meaning practice staff leave around a good supply of magazines to read for those who may, and often do, have a long wait. The problem with reading is that when you find something really interesting you become so absorbed in the details that you miss out on 'hearing' your name being called. It is of little use opting not to read in order to stay on the alert since boredom may set in and you could fall asleep.

Regular patients may be able to rely on being recognised by the reception staff who will make sure that they know when their name is called out. This can backfire when a new or temporary receptionist is on duty, particularly if her voice is too soft to be heard above the din of a children's play area in full cry. A good GP, on recognising the name on the file on his or her desk, will enlist the aid of a search party from the staff to track down his patient if the waiting has gone on for some time. If all else fails he may even come out of his consulting room in person to rescue his patient from the mental torture of the waiting-room.

Hospital departments and clinics make use of the ear symbol stickers issued through the Sympathetic Hearing scheme. The idea of using these is to help staff to be aware that the patient needs to be spoken to clearly or take more time over giving instructions. A sticker will only be placed on the hospital file if the patient has made it clear prior to the appointment that he or she is deaf or hard of hearing. Unfortunately there are some problems with the operation of this system.

Staff changes make it difficult for any establishment or organisation to keep up with the need for regular Deaf Awareness training and hospitals are no exception. A patient's file will not always be to hand as he is passed along the reception and treatments chain, the ear-graphics sticker may not be noticed and those who do see it may not understand its significance.

Most doctors and clinic staff rarely encounter people who are deaf or otherwise disabled, unless they work in a specialist clinic, and few will have received much if any Deaf Awareness training. As a consequence instructions can be difficult to follow.

Busy medical and nursing staff do not always look up in between writing their notes. Nor will they remember to pause while preparing a treatment and turn round to face you when speaking. When they do remember it is not always convenient for them to move or change position during a diagnosis or administering clinical treatment. Over the years successful writers of comedy situations have acquired some of their best ideas from observing the misunderstandings that can arise in this way. Things like surgical masks, essential for hygiene reasons, make it impossible to lip-read what the wearer is saying and the only answer may be to have the confidence before treatment starts to suggest a few simple signs or gestures that will convey instructions accurately. Without doubt patience and a sense of humour by both parties are helpful qualities at times like this.

Interpreters for the deaf will accompany a patient when attending doctors and dentists surgeries, and clinics or hospital appointments, if arranged in advance of the appointment. This does not necessarily mean that they have to be there, some individuals have more confidence than others in dealing with such situations by themselves.

For some clinical treatments a deaf person really does need to hang on to his sense of humour as well as what is left of his dignity. Being asked to lay face downwards and to keep very still can make it almost impossible to lip-read instructions and difficult to use any form of sign language. It can a pleasing experience for the men, though, if a pretty young nurse has been stationed at the 'head' end of the treatment couch - all that delightful eye and hand contact so close by!

The staff can be a bit less sympathetic in the Physiotherapy clinic. After all they are there purely to attend to your physical well-being. The mental aspect will come later once they are satisfied that their choice of treatment has worked.

Hearing-aid users can make themselves quite ill with the worry of deciding whether or not to switch off the hearing aid prior to treatment. One lady had an unforgettable experience during treatment for an injured ankle, wrists, and hands. The electronic equipment being used to treat the ankle was causing interference to her hearing-aid because she had forgotten to switch it off before treatment began. Left alone in a cubicle with both hands encased in warm wax and towels she could do nothing about it. It took another physiotherapist, looking in to investigate the source of the buzzing and beeping noises, to sort out the problem. She had to have it patiently explained to her how to switch off the hearing-aid. By which time, of course, the original physiotherapist had returned and wanted to know what all the fuss was about. She was not best pleased.

A visit to the dentist may be just as fraught. Profoundly deaf people without any hearing never experience the trauma of the high-pitched noise of a dentist's drill but trying to communicate during uncomfortable moments through their usual method of sign language can bring its own set of problems. Nevertheless the inability to hear unpleasant noises may help to reduce the level of stress that some dental treatments may otherwise raise.

The one place where hearing-aid users never have to worry about switching off the aid is when at the opticians. Instead, their problems, just as with those who rely upon some form of sign language, begin at the eyesight testing stage. Successful lip-reading becomes rather difficult to achieve when sitting in a darkened examination room and without the reassurance of those old and familiar spectacles to help. It is of little use asking the ophthalmologist, or whoever is carrying out the test, to write things down. Not only because the hand-written instructions may be illegible - as on so many medicine prescriptions - but the very reason for needing to have an eyesight test may make it difficult to read words.

For those who rely upon a recognised form of sign language to communicate they may find themselves having to teach a few key words and phrases before the test begins. If this is not sorted out beforehand then the test results may prove disastrous, and possibly expensive to put right.

A hospital stay is a traumatic experience for most people, not least for those who are deaf or hard-of-hearing who will have to cope with the additional problems created by poor communication. Visitors and interpreters can be a welcome presence in those situations. Patients who are allowed to be up and about may find others, whether walking or bed-bound, with whom they can communicate naturally and at ease - a benefit to both parties.

By making an extra effort to look after our health and persevering with those appointments for regular health-checks we will not only feel much better as a result but may make a valuable contribution to the furthering of deaf awareness.

CHAPTER TWELVE

GOOD HEALTH

Experts are constantly telling us what is and is not good for our health. Too much eating, or too little, how much to drink, how much sleep we should get, to exercise or not, smoking may bad for us - and then we are told that all things can be taken in moderation. That last statement sounds the most sensible, and the least confusing!

A hearing-impaired person especially should maintain a good level of health and strength to cope with the daily problems of communication. Particularly important is the need for regular amounts of sleep and exercise, a sensible diet and avoiding too much stress.

Stress can take many forms. Marriage is said to be one of them but so is divorce. The birth of a child is another, and the shock of a bereavement. Moving house can be traumatic, so can changing jobs. Then there are those situations that arise from a series of family crises or problems at work, or imprisonment for whatever reason. How we cope with any of these mostly unavoidable situations depends much on our individual strengths and weaknesses.

There are other causes of stress that can be avoided or reduced. The worst culprit being excessive noise. Too much of this will damage our hearing. Even for the profoundly deaf their sense of awareness or touch will feel strong sound-vibrations sent out from the source of extreme noise. Unfortunately because sound-waves are invisible we may be unaware of the damage being caused to our hearing until years later. And then it will be too late to do anything about it.

The louder the noise is, the longer we are exposed to it, the greater the risk.

How can we tell?

Try talking, without shouting, to someone who is standing about two metres away.

You can hear each other? Fine.

Now try it where there is a lot of background noise going on.

More difficult, isn't it? That means the noise is approaching danger level.

Noise levels are measured in dBA, a decibel scale that reflects the sensitivity of human ears to different pitches of sound:

20 dBA is a quiet room at night;

40 dBA is a quiet sitting room;

60 dBA is ordinary spoken conversation;

80 dBA is shouting;

110 dBA is a pneumatic drill nearby;

130 dBA is an aeroplane taking off 100 metres away;

140 dBA is the threshold of pain.

In other words all sounds over 80 dBA can damage your ears. Loud noise is a feature of everyday life but not all of it has to be endured. It would be lovely if someone could invent noiseless traffic on our roads and pneumatic drills, power tools and machinery that sang sweetly instead of threatening to split our ear-drums. We all have our dreams.

A lot of people enjoy following their television and radio programmes with the sound system turned up at full volume. As already pointed out, this is quite unnecessary for those who can use a loop system to hear through or have a television displaying Teletext and/or subtitling. Those with normal hearing who persist in listening with the volume turned up do themselves no favours. They not only cause frayed tempers with their neighbours but permanent damage to their own hearing.

At the cinema there are occasions when the film soundtrack can be too loud. The obvious person to complain to is the cinema manager - especially if he sees you wearing a pair of ear protectors. True, he might take umbrage and refuse to co-operate but just think of the publicity your cause would receive if the story ended up in the local newspaper.

Wearing proper ear protectors or having ear plugs handy are a help in all kinds of situations. You only have to see the number of photographs and film-shots taken to realise just how often these are worn by those trained to handle and use firearms and explosives. If more young people were to protect their ears in this way when at discos then there would be less instances of early deafness. An obvious alternative to wearing such protectors would be to avoid being near the source of noise in the first place but not everyone likes to be thought of as unsociable.

At work there are laws, called the Noise at Work Regulations, that aim to protect our hearing and all employers should follow the Management of Health and Safety at Work Regulations. These bind them to have noise levels assessed and to keep a record of those assessments. If daily noise levels reach or exceed 85 dBA the employer must let you know about the risks and explain how to protect your ears. He must also provide ear protectors and keep them in good repair. Every effort should be made to reduce noise levels as far as possible by modifying or replacing equipment and maintaining it regularly. Where the daily level is above 90dBA ear protectors must be worn. Areas where these have to be worn they should be clearly marked as Ear Protection Zones. If this is a regular part of the daily work routine then the employer must arrange for your hearing to be tested regularly by experts and to keep records of the test results. He should make sure that these results are given to you and that you receive medical advice if there is hearing loss.

Stress management is a recognised way of handling the many forms of stress, including those associated with a hearing loss.

Suffering from vertigo, or dizziness, is one example of a stressful situation. Most people feel dizzy at some point in their lives, from all sorts of causes. Children, for instance, will spin round and round for the sheer fun of making themselves giddy. If you move your head suddenly you may feel dizzy. So does taking too many fairground rides or drinking too much alcohol. Certain kinds of travel may also cause this sensation.

Conditions such as vertigo caused by a health-related problem may be helped in all sorts of ways - medication, surgery, exercises, a change of spectacles or simply relaxing in a warm bath instead of rushing to take a quick shower.

Regular exercises, as those instructed by professionally trained people, help to keep limbs and body supple as will gentle massaging. The hands and neck are particularly susceptible to arthritic conditions and those who rely on lip-reading need to be able to turn the head often and freely, without pain. Hands and fingers need to be kept flexible if you are dependent upon using the hand and finger alphabet for communicating. The British Sign Language (BSL) in particular ideally requires mobile hand, arm and body movements.

Yoga classes are a good way to exercise and maintain that flexibility but remember to position yourself where you can watch what is happening. If you relax too much and close your eyes you are likely to miss out on what you should do next - unless you are a genius at lip-reading with your eyes shut.

Aerobic classes may be good for physical fitness but any music played at full volume to accompany it is likely to seriously damage your hearing if not your wealth.

There are a number of medical conditions which, as with dizziness, can lead to a loss of balance whether temporary or permanent. There are special exercises - the Cawthorne-Cooksey exercises - that retrain your balance system by giving your brain practice with the new balance signals it is receiving. As you do the exercises you make all sorts of simple movements in every position. It is best to do them exactly as taught by a physiotherapist or other qualified practitioner with experience of helping in this way. The exercises will be worked out for you to practice at your own pace so that you do not make yourself feel sick or dizzy. They do need to be done regularly over a period of several weeks to achieve a good result.

The sense of loneliness and isolation that deafness can bring may induce its own form of stress and it is very important to learn how to override it. Contact with other human beings is important for mental welfare and even the most reserved of individuals should make some effort to mix with society, even if it is just a weekly visit to the shops.

For the housebound deaf who are able use a telephone in whatever specially adapted form this is the next best means of contact as is the increasing use of the home computer. Overuse, though, can bring its own problems.

Lengthy phone calls by a textphone user may end with aching wrists, stiff fingers, eye strain or all three. Constant sitting in front of personal computers (PCs) will cause eye-strain as well as aching backs, necks, arms and hands. Hearing-aid telephone users can end up with a bruised ear from sandwiching it between the hearing-aid and the telephone receiver for too long. As for those who think they can manage perfectly well with the hands-free fashion of gripping the receiver between the neck and the shoulder they may end up not only with a sore neck and pains between the shoulders but can, according to recent medical research, create a hidden timebomb of serious health problems for the future such as blocking the flow of blood through one or both arteries in the neck.

Blood circulatory problems cause dizziness and loss of balance, as does an excess of caffeine consumption, nicotine or alcohol. Cutting down on the latter group is believed to reduce the instances of migraine, tinnitus and the attacks of giddiness which occur with Menière's Disease. Deciding what to do for best in these situations is seldom easy.

It is well-known that when one sense is lost others develop to compensate that loss. As a general example the blind develop a keener sense of hearing, and touch will become more sensitive. The deaf may become more visually aware, be more sensitive to vibrations and their sense of smell more keen.

None of these senses can be relied upon alone since apart from their being dependent on other physical conditions the brain has to be reasonably alert to cope with recognising the messages received. This is one good reason for trying to keep to a regular sleeping pattern and making use of relaxation techniques and advice.

Strong smells dominate, of course, which is useful when there is a gas leak or something is burning but not so much fun when out on a country walk and passing the local sewage treatment works. They may also mask smells that would otherwise give warning of danger. Cigarette smoke, for example, will mask the kind of smells that a hearing person would link with the hissing of a leaking gas pipe or tap, the crackling or spitting of an electrical fire, or liquids boiling over on the kitchen stove.

For the deaf and hearing alike it is important that the ears should be kept clean and regularly checked for wax deposits building up in the ear canal. Never poke anything into the ears - unless they are prescribed eardrops or earplugs. That action may push down further any wax which is already there. Cotton-wool buds leave behind tiny fibres which can irritate the ear membrane and fingers or towels may damage the skin and carry infection.

Ear-cleaning must be done under strict medical supervision to avoid damaging the hearing. The practice nurse at the local GP's surgery is trained to syringe ears and will do so once the few drops of oil first applied have been given time to work through the ear canal and softened the wax. The problem with syringing with water, apart from the mess, is that if the jet of liquid is forced too hard it may damage the ear. A recommended method of removing ear wax is with the use of a probe by the doctor but this is an acquired skill and needs a lot of practice. An Ear Nose and Throat (ENT) specialist can take up to six months to learn and develop the skill required, whereas a general practitioner (GP) rarely sees a patient requiring ear-cleaning and would take far longer to learn the technique.

Both methods can cause some discomfort. Syringing, even when a specially shaped dish is pressed close against the neck to catch the water spillage, can result in a tedious mopping up operation. A probe can feel uncomfortable as it is pushed deeper into the ear canal but since no water is used the clothes, and the patient, stay dry. It should be the only method to be used with people suffering from Menière's Disease.

Ears should also be checked at the first sign of unexplained discomfort or pain, especially if they have recently been in contact with dirty water. This may carry bacteria that can cause an infection and which may block your ear temporarily - a good reason for ensuring that ears are dried out thoroughly after washing your hair. Public swimming pools in the UK are generally well maintained but pools in foreign holiday resorts may not be so. Hearing-aid wearers should make sure that ear-moulds are wiped clean with a soft cloth before storing away.

When we do need medical advice and obtain prescription drugs it is important that a chemist checks that the information given for prescribed drug treatment is properly understood. The label on the container must be clearly written and include all essential instructions. The chemist should ensure that when these are read out he/she speaks clearly and is properly understood. Some harassed counter assistants have been known to shout at and cause a lot of personal embarrassment to the customer/patient. For those taking medication there are a choice of pill organisers to make sure that tablets are taken at the prescribed times.

Far too much publicity is given to diets and weightwatching for it to be necessary to include these topics in this book. Healthy eating will help to keep our senses more alert and to feel less stressed. For those who take their weight-watching seriously there are a range of bathroom scales suitable for all users including Brailled ones for those with little or no sight. Suffice it to say that the less weight we carry around the more active we can be, and able to bend down to pick up that dropped hearing-aid battery.

CHAPTER THIRTEEN

HOBBIES AND INTERESTS

Few hobbies and interests are off limits to the deaf or hearing-impaired. With a little bit of perseverance it is possible for people of mixed abilities to meet and socialise together in pursuit of a favourite pastime. With a few exceptions there should be no need for the segregation of those with physical and sensory abilities as has been the pattern in the past.

As mentioned earlier a deaf learner car driver can have more fun than a hearing one. The learner will quickly discover that he can feel the vibrations of the engine changes when his feet are resting on the foot controls. As a result he is often ready to change gears before the poor instructor has finished working out how to explain this in some form sign language! Another advantage is the extra visual skill this driver has developed, so useful in anticipating the changes that occur during driving. Unfortunately, this superior knowledge is not always appreciated by instructors and so is best used as tactfully as possible.

The popularity of Nature-watching is increasing as a leisure pursuit. Not only does it give an opportunity to take some healthy exercise out of doors but has the added bonus of watching wildlife on the move. As any enthusiast will tell us, the visual side of this is only part of the story. The sounds that the creatures make can be fascinating to listen to and using a portable cassette recorder is an ideal way to record them. They can be played back at a sound volume to suit. Bird-watchers - that is those 'twitchers' who watch the feathered variety - should beware of playing back the tape on the spot or they will have a chorus of birds singing back to their own tape recorded voices.

These days changing natural habitats mean that you may not need to go far from home if regular visitors such as foxes, hedgehogs or frogs adopt your garden, or the neighbours'. The snuffling sounds of hedgehogs as they rummage around in search of food may sound amusing but the constant croaking of frogs in their 'happy' season can be downright irritating to those with normal hearing. Those who have never heard these fascinating noises can become a pain in the neck to their nearest and dearest with their pleading to record those sounds. They will be wise to remember, if their plea is successful, to use personal headphones before they play back the recording at a volume to suit them best or the outcome may be a smashed cassette-player or tape recorder.

Learn to play a musical instrument? Why not? Piano playing and any musical instrument that uses percussion, such as drums, give out wonderful vibrations. You do not need to be able to hear sound when you can enjoy the feel of the rhythm. There are concerts given and cassettes and books are available on the theme of Fun With Music.

Specialist interests such as collecting coins, postcards or stamps are quiet and absorbing hobbies. They are ideal for those who are profoundly deaf but can all too easily become solitary occupations. Likewise are interests that require nimble fingers and endless patience such as model-making. The way to get the best satisfaction from hobbies of this kind is to make use of the need to build on the collection and thus explore new avenues. Problems can arise when communicating with dealers or attending meetings but most people are only too happy to help and make contact with fellow enthusiasts on an equal footing.

For those deafblind but with residual sight it may be possible to use a specially adapted magnifier or a spectacle-mounted telescope to aid reading or inspecting details more clearly. This applies to any hobby or specialist interest requiring attention to its finer points. There are various writing guides to choose from that will help to keep lines straight and the writing neat for those who have to put together presentation notes for any talks they may be invited to give.

A needle threader is a boon to most craftworkers and for those with little or no eyesight a specially embossed tape measure, knitting needle gauge or knitting clock is so useful.

Furniture-making can be fraught with dangers for most people and very taxing on their reserves of patience. For the deafblind trying to glue pieces together the right way up or round, the charity swearbox may swell from a sizeable monetary contribution. Some would say that this applies to any fool who thinks he can do better than a trained craftsman.

Except, possibly, for those suffering from Menière's disease where the sense of balance can be badly affected, learning to dance is an interest that can be attempted by all. Tripping the light fantastic can take many forms, not just gyrating at discos but Country and Barn dancing, tap, ballet, Modern, Old-time, Ballroom, Latin American, and many others. Dancers do need to maintain good posture and footwork in order to move smoothly through each dance step and this can only be achieved by practice. People talk about dancing with two left feet but if the body and mind is relaxed through the confidence gained from learning the steps properly there will be less likelihood of loss of balance.

Lip-reading can be a useful asset when dancing - both at the dance itself and at lessons. The music may well be too loud for 'hearing' dancers to try holding a conversation but not for the deaf - unless they attempt to reply at length using sign language while cavorting around the dance-floor. The keen deaf dancer uses the technique of remembering and counting the timing of the steps as a substitute to following the sound of the music. This can create a slight problem, called memory lapse, when the partner interrupts with some comment that has to be hastily lip-read. The lack of concentration can result in painful physical contact with toes or knees. Learning a Latin American dance, such as the Cha-cha-cha, can create misunderstandings. One deaf pupil took a long time to realise that a 'Turkish Tail' was 'Turkish Towel', and that an 'Aida' was not the cue to burst into a rendering from the famous opera.

Most dance teachers are good communicators, ready to describe new dance steps by almost any means, a skill much-appreciated by the deaf and hearing alike. They are equally adept at ducking and diving to avoid arms outflung in the attempt to compensate for that sudden loss of balance.

For more outgoing people with some ability to communicate with the hearing world, sports activities present few problems. For a deaf person who has had little or no close contact with hearing people this may be more difficult. When poor speaking ability makes it hard for hearing people to understand them it can be very discouraging for those who do want to join in.

Most deaf clubs have interests the same as hearing clubs and thus a profoundly deaf person may prefer to join the former instead. Competitive sporting opportunities are lost when these clubs, because of their smaller size, do not have enough members to cover, say, a football team. Much talent and enthusiasm has been lost because of these problems and attitudes. This is a great pity for since 1969 the Olympic Committee has officially recognised the status of World Games for the Deaf. As if to prove a point, in that same year, at Belgrade, deaf British athletes between them collected medals which included two golds, one silver and one bronze.

Deaf people can be sports coaches for the deaf and hearing alike - an asset when required to mediate as an interpreter for explaining techniques and practice methods. Many more are needed if sporting talents are to be used to the full. Likewise there is plenty of room for more deaf awareness advice and training to be given at sports clubs and through other sporting links.

Hearing-aids are of invaluable help to many but until technology overcomes all the drawbacks of using them it will always be a good idea to acquire additional skills in lip-reading. This, combined with looking, thinking and listening, helps in communicating more freely. Looking means observing the whole person for body language and facial expressions as well as speech movements. Thinking means learning to anticipate and follow the gist of conversation. Listening means hearing sounds that may seem distorted or incomplete until matched with the shape of the mouth, as formed with speech movements, to make greater word sense.

Lip-reading tutors are a valuable source of information and will help with improving and developing your lip-reading skills. They will also advise on ways to cope with difficult hearing situations and on the support services available to people with impaired hearing.

A Lip-reading Class is a small informal and friendly group made up of people with similar problems who learn not only about hearing-aids but about which other aids might best help overcome the day to day difficulties faced at home, at work and in leisure time.

Attendance at a lip-reading class can help rebuild some of the confidence lost through deafness whilst providing the opportunity for self-help, mutual support and friendship with people who understand those problems.

Organisations and local charities that have strong links with deaf people, such as the RAD, arrange many courses designed to help make communication easier. Advice and coaching in signing and sign language skills is available to allcomers, both deaf and hearing alike. They are also behind much of the work involved with the Deaf Awareness training advice given out to local businesses and the community at large. All this in addition to providing social clubs where the deaf and hard of hearing can meet to exchange gossip and ideas.

Trained Interpreters have now made it possible for deaf people to enjoy the theatre. They stand at the side of the stage so that the deaf person can watch the production being performed and see the information being described by the interpreter at the same time. They are also present at key conferences held at national events - allowing deaf and hearing-aid users to participate on equal terms with the hearing audiences and delegates.

There are many deaf, and deafblind, who have a natural ability to teach skills to others and there are many practical activities from which to choose. The range can include the simple, such as craft-work, knitting, or needlework, to the more complex like dancing, woodworking, practical electronics, computer programming or cooking. The deafblind, through the use of adapted Brailled or marked equipment, are particularly adept at playing and teaching games of chess, draughts, Scrabble, dominoes, cards, and many other board games

It does take patience to teach but once achieved it is so very rewarding.

Last, but not least, is the role of escorting others with greater or different disabilities to places of interest. It is also a means of enabling them to participate in sports activities or at a club meeting. The arrangements made do not have to be frequent or time-consuming but they are an ideal way to meet different people and exploring new ground.

Learning more about other interests in this way can become quite addictive!

CHAPTER FOURTEEN

ENTERTAINMENT AND SOCIAL LIFE

Social events bring problems as well as enjoyment.

For hearing-aid wearers the aid may stop functioning, such as when the battery runs down - usually at the most inconvenient times. At the theatre, for example, it can be very frustrating to have spent an hour or more following the excitement of a good drama only for your hearing-aid to fail just before the curtain is due to fall and you miss the cliff-hanger ending. On the other hand if there is a scene in which the villain of the piece pulls out a gun then a hearing-aid battery is sure to wait until after the noise of the firing has died down before it runs out. You may well think that the shooting has destroyed the sound system when a wall of silence hits you. It is only when you see the rest of the audience clapping their hands that you realise it is your aid that needs urgent attention.

Similar problems can occur at the cinema and not just because the darkened auditorium makes it difficult to see which way up the new hearing-aid battery should go into its drawer. Trying to find it and retrieve from under someone else's seat if you drop it on the floor may be regarded as unacceptable social behaviour. As pointed out in an earlier chapter the enjoyment of the film can be marred by the volume being too loud, and the sound quality is not always as good as it should be. It may also be spoilt by the reaction of others when you are heard to complain.

The best appreciated dramas, on film or in the theatre, are those relying upon acting and miming with a minimum of dialogue but these are few and far between. Professional film makers and producers of stage dramas have yet to receive training in deaf awareness.

But why go out? Why not avoid mixing with people and stay at home? Well, why not? We are all free to do as we please, up to a point. It is not only the deaf or hearing-impaired who may have a fear or dislike of venturing out socially. A surprising number of those with full hearing think that way too. Not everyone is blessed, or cursed, with confidence or has an extrovert personality. Of those who do live with someone who is like that there may be times when they perhaps wish that things could be otherwise.

Not everyone is bothered about meeting someone who would make an ideal partner for sharing his or her life. Some are perfectly happy to remain completely independent of others all their lives. It is a fact, though, that deafness can limit one's chances of meeting such a partner, if they are seeking one. By how much those chances are reduced is down to the amount of effort made by the individual.

There is a lot of truth that going to a dance is a good way of achieving this aim. For those happy to mix socially then the time and effort spent on taking a few dance lessons beforehand can bring its own reward. Indeed, many dance studios and teachers run social evenings where those with a common interest in trying out new dance steps can meet and practice together. All that eye contact for lip-reading, hands and fingers touching plus lots of opportunities for miming practice not only produce some interesting reactions but can be a lot of fun.

The majority of pastimes and interests are centred on visual display and meetings and major events such as air shows and theme parks can be enjoyed almost as much as without hearing any accompanying commentary. Deaf people are natural observers and will notice all kinds of additional incidents and individual touches that give a richness and colour to what is happening around them. There is no need for them to worry if they cannot hear the aeroplanes flying overhead. They will know when a lot of noise is being made when they see a small child flapping its hands against its ears as it plays at receiving and shutting out the sounds.

As previously pointed out background noises can be very distracting for the hearing-aid user when trying to follow a conversation. Those deaf who rely upon signing are in the habit of forming a circle when meeting socially so that all hand movements and facial expressions can be read clearly. Without this arrangement a deaf person will not know, or cannot be sure, if they are being spoken to. It is a practice which all should try to follow but is not always possible when meeting in crowded places such as pubs, theatre and cinema foyers, or restaurants. The frequent shifting of positions and jostling, as well as any background noise, makes it difficult to keep up with the changing topics during a conversation. A person relying upon a mix of hearing and lip-reading to follow a discussion needs to be in a central position to pick up key words and short sentences to help make a sensible contribution to the general talk.

It is not generally realised that the condition known as colour blindness is a hindrance to lip-reading ability. A lip-reader needs colour to aid recognition of mouth shapes, which is one reason why colour television has been such a helpful invention. Special contact lenses have been developed which help to compensate colour blindness.

Invitations to dinner can be fraught with all kinds of problems - and not just the worry of what to wear or finding a reliable baby-sitter. Candle-lit meals, and side lights around the room can make it almost impossible to see clearly enough for lip-reading. So can trying to eat at the same time as someone is speaking. Often the food ends up being speared by guesswork while continuing to look at the face of the speaker and what was a hot meal soon becomes cold. And, since we all know that it is rude to speak with one's mouth full, trying to respond sensibly and promptly may prove to be rather embarrassing. It can put you right off your meal when your find yourself lip-reading someone who is speaking before they have swallowed a mouthful of food - or worse, with the fork or spoon still jutting from the bottom lip.

If several people are sitting around the table and more than one of them is talking then it is difficult to know which face to look at in order to follow any sort of conversation. For the experienced lip-reader it is often easier, and sometimes more interesting, to follow what is being discussed at the far end of the table. The only trouble with this arrangement is that you will catch the unsuspecting speakers by surprise when you attempt to join in - if they are able to hear you. For conversations closer to hand it is demoralising when a well-intentioned person takes over answering on a deaf person's behalf.

Eating out at barbecues or other outdoor parties brings its own set of problems. How can you use your hands for signing or sign language when you are holding a plate of food or a wine or beer glass? Then there is the difficulty, as the daylight fails and low wattage safety or patio lights are switched on, of trying to lip-read or follow signing movements masked by the evening's shadows. If you opt out of going to these events then you run the risk of being regarded as anti-social. On the other hand if you do attend but stay quietly in the background this may be interpreted either as being shy or downright rude. It can be a no-win situation. The best way around the problem is to latch on to someone who enjoys being listened to and does so noisily - not every party visitor is boring and you might even learn something new.

For the deaf and hearing alike there are concerts to enjoy which use signing or sign language simultaneously with the music and singing. At concert halls where loop and infrared systems are available the hearing-aid user can enjoy the music being played almost as well as those with normal hearing. This does though rather depend on the quality and range of the sound system in use. Concerts that include musical instruments which give out strong pulsing vibrations when played are particularly appreciated - these are likely to include the piano, xylophone, drum, or wind instrument in particular. But, unless you are completely deaf, be careful to avoid excessive noise entering the ear while experimenting with the volume control on whichever assistive aid is used, or with the hearing aid itself.

Had enough of going out and want to stay at home for a change? Then how about putting on a videoed film with subtitles to watch? The local library will happily loan you a few. Not only that but they can even offer some that will help you brush up on your knowledge of fingerspelling and sign language - ready for the next time you venture out.

CHAPTER FIFTEEN

TRAVEL AND HOLIDAYS

There are any number of problems encountered with travel when using public transport whether it be by rail, bus, coach, boat, or 'plane. Some of them can be overcome whilst others, just as for the travelling public in general, simply have to be endured.

All main terminals used for public transport have loudspeaker or Tannoy systems which are used for the various announcements needed to be made. They are also installed in public service road vehicles, trains and chartered transport used for long distance travel, such as coaches, boats and aeroplanes. The sound quality of these systems, combined with poor acoustic conditions, can make it difficult even for people with normal hearing to understand what is being said. This is a problem which travellers have had to endure ever since Tannoy systems were first installed. Hence the old joke that they are there 'tannoya'!

Not only are there problems with mishearing announcements but in places where visual alternatives, such as indicator boards, may not always work as well as they should. Extensive use of visual display units and other forms of information displays using digital technology are replacing these.

As a direct result of the rapid expansion of international travel many improvements are being made in the field of communications. The particular problems created when visitors arrive at their foreign destinations with insufficient knowledge of the local language have brought about greater awareness of the need to communicate more efficiently and quickly. Airports use plenty of visual aids including many picture type symbols and graphics that are much appreciated by international travellers. One possible problem from this increase in ease of international travelling is that some may have difficulty in deciding at which airport they have arrived. Unlike railway, bus or boat services, place names are not usually the first thing which flight passengers see as their plane touches down at an airport terminal.

For the deafblind there is much help available for getting themselves out and about independently of others. There are simple but effective canes to use, the simplest is a white cane with red bands. Modern technology has produced a Mowat Sensor that is an ultra-sonic torch that vibrates when objects come within its beam - a handy location device.

With the coming of space exploration a rash of orbiting satellites have appeared, receiving and sending all kinds of information through signals beamed to their receiving stations on the ground below. Through such signals and the series of sensors placed alongside the roads it is now possible to have battery-operated bleeper alert systems for planning road travel and so avoid traffic-congested areas. The same technology, used in easily portable form, can be used to guide blind or partially sighted walkers safely along their way.

The development of digital technology has also made large print and tactile maps more easily available. And for walking in towns textured paving has been created to indicate the location of pelican or zebra crossings.

We all need a holiday from time to time to renew the energy we need to cope with the daily round of problems that our lives may bring.

For the less well-off, caravans and self-catering places are usually an inexpensive way to holiday away from home in reasonable comfort. They can be ideal for those wishing to get away from the crowds. Less so, though, if the caravan turns out to be in the middle of a busy holiday camping site when the brochure illustrations clearly showed an open field. There can be problems when things like the water supply does not work properly, or worse, neither do the sanitation arrangements. Then there are those times when a heavy downpour of rain threatens to wash the whole area away in a sea of mud. The caravan can have the electricity supply cut off or damaged if it is part of an established site. Cooking plans can be ruined if the gas stove stops working or the supply of bottled gas suddenly runs out.

What has all this to do with being deaf?

A great deal if you are holidaying alone and need to communicate with others when help is urgently needed. The nearest inhabited place is certain to be lived in by a hermit or someone unwilling or with little patience to understand the problem. At times like these a few hearing companions to share the holiday are much appreciated. The downside of that arrangement is having to put up with them complaining about the noise of the rain lashing down on the caravan roof. To them it may sound like several hundred marbles crashing down over their heads - especially if they have been out sampling the local beer or scrumpy the night before.

Staying in strange places such as hotels or guest-houses set up in converted old buildings can be disconcerting for all kinds of reasons if holidaying alone. Most wearers of hearing-aids prefer to remove them at night in order to get a comfortable night's sleep. This innocent act may create all sorts of problems to the hotel or guest house staff if their 'guest' cannot be woken up for whatever reason. Of course the room door can be left unlocked overnight to allow for unforeseen emergencies but there is the risk of this action being misconstrued by some guests. It could also prove to be an embarrassing disaster for the inebriated or absentminded who may enter the wrong room by mistake.

The alternative of trying to sleep with the hearing-aid switched on may turn out to be nerve-wracking experience. Apart from the physical discomfort of the aid being squashed between a rock hard pillow and the side of the head, trying to remain in a semi-conscious state of alertness throughout the night in anticipation of unexpected intruders can be a frightening experience. There are so many strange and unrecognisable noises to be heard. Unfamiliar sounds such as the creaking of old timber joists, the rattling of ancient chimney pots and raindrops spattering against the windows can have the nervous diving deep beneath the bedclothes or even under the bed itself.

And what of those to whom sound means nothing or very little?

Who has never been afraid of the shadows of the night?

Film-making companies have made small fortunes from creating stories developed from terrifying situations such as these.

Holiday destinations need not be confined to one country where the native language is in daily use. In fact there are times when it can be easier to understand a foreign language than the local dialect of the home country.

These days because of the rapid spread of the English language through the dominating American influence on computer systems there is less need to acquire an extensive vocabulary of a foreign language before travelling abroad. This may apply not only to those who prefer to restrict their holiday pleasures to the Costa del Sol, but for those seeking greater adventures further afield.

This is all very well but think how much more interesting a foreign holiday could be were we to take the trouble to learn more about the local people and their language. The French are known to complain bitterly about the way some of their compatriots have adopted English words to use as part of their daily life. For the car traveller abroad this can work in his or her favour when they discover that the word *parking* is recognised in both countries for the same purpose. And the word *stop!* is used in many countries on traffic-warning signs, useful for emergency situations.

The one thing in common between those who use forms of sign language to help them communicate and the local people in other countries is their natural ability to use body and hand language to express themselves more clearly. This is in addition to the existence of the official international sign language of Gestuno.

For those with enough hearing to try learning new words and pronunciations things can be a little more difficult, but not impossible. A little extra thought on how best to achieve the right results, some perseverance and plenty of practice will go a long way to mastering this new skill. The achievement will give confidence to travel further afield and thus acquire a greater understanding of our neighbours and make new friendships.

Remember, none of us was put on this earth to live alone nor to take things easy but to work together as a part of a community. Man was a hunter long before he settled to live in entrenched dwellings but his instinct to survive is still there. The deaf and the deafblind have to work harder than most to ensure acceptance by the hearing members of the community. By their very example they show how this can be done - through patience, tolerance and, above all, their sense of humour. They have to in order to survive!

Name and Contact details (UNITED KINGDOM)

BDA (British Deaf Association)
1 - 3 Worship Street,
London, EC2A 2AB
Tel (voice): *020 7588 3529*
Fax: *020 7588 3527*
Textphone: *020 7588 3529*
Website: www.britishdeafassociation.org.uk
The largest U.K. organisation run by deaf people for deaf people.

Regional office - north-west England:
33 Wilson Patten Street,
Warrington,
Lancashire, WA1 1PG
Tel (voice): *019 2565 2520*
Fax: *019 2565 2526*
Textphone *019 2565 2529*

Northern Ireland office:
Suite 3, Cranmore House,
611b Lisburn Road,
Belfast, BT9 7GT
Tel (voice) *028 9038 7700*
Fax: *028 9038 7707*
Textphone: *028 9038 7706*
Videophone: *028 9038 2677*

Scotland office:
Princes House, 3rd Floor,
5 Shandwick Place
Edinburgh, EH2 4RG
Tel (voice): *013 1221 2600*
Fax: *013 1229 4067*
Textphone: *013 1229 3833*

Wales office:
Shand House,
2 Fitzalan Place,
Cardiff, CF24 0BE
Tel (voice) *029 2030 2216*
Fax: *029 2030 2218*
Textphone: *029 2030 2217*

CACDP (Council for the Advancement of Communication with Deaf People)
Durham University Science Park
Block 4, Stockton Road,
Durham, DH1 3UZ
Tel: *0191 383 1155*
Fax: *0191 383 7914*
Textphone: *0191 383 7915*
Website: www.cacdp.org.uk
Offers nationally recognised examinations in British Sign Language and other forms of communication used by deaf people. It also works to ensure deaf people have access to the same rights - social, economic and legal, as hearing people.

CACDP Northern Ireland office:
Wilton House,
5 College Square North
Belfast, BT 6AR
Tel., Fax and
Textphone: *(028) 90 438 161*

CACDP Scotland office:
123/129 High Street
Glasgow, G1 1PH
Tel: *0141 559 5366*
Fax and Textphone: *0141 559 5367*

Defeating Deafness
The Hearing Research Trust
330-332 Gray's Inn Road
London, WC1X 8EE
Tel: 020 7833 1733
Fax: 020 7278 0404
Textphone: 020 7915 1412
Website: www.defeatingdeafness.org
Supports research into the diagnosis, prevention, treatment and cure of hearing difficulties.

Hearing Concern
4th Floor,
275-281 King Street
London, W6 9LZ
Tel: 020 8233 2929
Fax and textphone: 020 8233 2934
Website: www.hearingconcern.com
Campaigns to raise public awareness of the needs and rights of hearing-impaired people and co-ordinates the Sympathetic Hearing Scheme.

HIYPE! (Hearing Impaired Young People)
(Website only)
Website: www.hiype.org.uk
The only website in the UK for hearing impaired people who are working or studying.

NDCS (National Deaf Children's Society)
15 Dufferin Street,
London EC1Y 8UR
Tel: 020 7490 8656
Fax: 020 7251 5020
Textphone: 0207490 8656
Website: www.ndcs.org.uk
Provides information, advice and support with aspects of childhood deafness. Full information and details of their offices in Belfast, Birmingham, Cardiff and Glasgow are on their website.

RAD (Royal Association for Deaf People)
Walsingham Road,
Colchester,
Essex, CO2 7BP
Tel: *01206 509509*
Fax: *01206 769755*
Textphone: *01206 711260*
Website: www.royaldeaf.org.uk
It endeavours to meet the needs of people affected by deafness and provide deaf awareness advice through its Centres in south-east England.

RNID (Royal National Institute for Deaf People)
19-23 Featherstone Street
London, EC1Y 8SL
Tel: *020 7296 8000*
Fax: *020 7296 8199*
Textphone: *020 7296 8001*
Website: www.rnid.org.co.uk
The largest U.K. charity providing a wide range of information, advice and support to deaf and hard-of-hearing people. For more information, and details of all their regional offices, visit their website.

Sense
11-13 Clifton Terrace,
London, N4 3SR
Tel: *020 7272 7774*
Fax: *0207272 6012*
Textphone: *020 7272 9648*
Website: www.sense.org.uk
Supports and campaigns for people who are both deaf and blind, their families, carers, and professionals who work with them.

The Menière's Society
98 Maybury Road,
Woking
Surrey, GU21 5HX
Tel: +44 (0) 1483 7405977
Fax: +44 (0) 1483 755441
Textphone +44 (0) 1483 771207
Website: www.menieres.co.uk
Provides advice and support to sufferers of Menière's Disease. Encourages the formation of local self-help groups and further research into the disease.

The British Tinnitus Association
Ground Floor, Unit 5, Acorn Business Park,
Woodseats Close,
Sheffield, S8 0TB
Tel: 0800 018 0527 free of charge (from within the U.K only)
Tel: 0845 4500 321 local rate (from within the U.K. only)
Tel: 0114 250 9922 national rate (within the U.K)
Tel: +44 (0)114 250 9922 (outside the U.K)
Fax: 0114 258 2279 (from within the U.K)
Fax: +44 (0)114 258 2279 (outside the U.K)
Textphone: 0114 258 5694 (from within the U.K)
Textphone: +44 (0)114 258 2279 (outside the U.K)
Website: www.tinnitus.org.uk
Provides advice, information and support and promotes further research into this condition.

Tinnitus Helpline - R.N.I.D.
Website: www.rnid.org.co.uk

Hearing Dogs for Deaf People
The Grange, Wycombe Road, Saunderton,
Princes Risborough,
Buckinghamshire, HP27 9NS
Tel. and Textphone: *01844 340 100*
Fax: *01844 348 101*
Trains and places hearing dogs with people who are deaf or hearing-impaired.

The Beatrice Wright Training Centre (part of Hearing Dogs for Deaf People)
Hull Road,
Cliffe, Selby,
North Yorkshire, YO8 6NG
Tel. and Textphone: *01757 638 666*
Fax: *01757 630 560*
Website: www.hearing-dogs.co.uk
Trains and places hearing dogs with people who are deaf or hearing-impaired.

Deaf Action (formerly known as Edinburgh & East of Scotland Deaf Society)
49 Albany Street,
Edinburgh, EH1 3QY
Tel: *0131 556 3128*
Fax: *0131 557 8283*
Textphone: *0131 557 0419*
Website: www.deafsociety.org
Works to provide services which meet the needs of those who are deaf

Visit the websites of organisations such as RNID or NCDS for full details of all regional offices and local contacts.

Name and Contact details (IRISH REPUBLIC)

Art & Cultural Society of the Deaf
40 Lower Drumcondra Road,
Dublin 9
Fax: *+353-1-285.80.92*
Website: www.iol.ie
Their aim is to promote Irish Deaf Culture at home and abroad.

Kerry Deaf Resource Centre
4 Gas Terrace,
Tralee,
Co. Kerry
Tel and Fax: *+353 66 712 0399*
Videophone: *+353 66 712 0386*
Website: www.kerrydeaf.com

Irish Hard of Hearing Association
Website: www.ihha.ie

Irish Tinnitus Association
Website: www.nadp.ie

National Association for Deaf People
Website: www.nadp.ie
note: The above three organisations share the same address and contact numbers:
35 North Frederick Street,
Dublin 1.
Tel/Textphone: *01 8723800*
Fax: *01 8723816*

Name and Contact details (UNITED STATES OF AMERICA)

ALDA (Association of Late-Deafened Adults)
1131 Lake St., # 204
Oak Park IL 60301
Phone (Voice)/Fax: *877-907-1738*
TTY: *708-358-0135*
Website: www.alda.org
Provides help and support to those who have been raised in the hearing world but became deaf later in life.

Alexander Graham Bell Association for the Deaf and Hard of Hearing
3417 Volta Place NW
NW Washington
DC 20007
Phone (Toll Free) *(866) 337-5220*
Phone: *(202) 337-5220*
TTY: *(202) 337-5221*
Fax: *(202) 337-8314*
Website: www.agbell.org/
The U.S.A's largest information and support center for pediatric hearing loss and oral/deaf education. It provides networking opportunities for those who are deaf or hard of hearing.

American Society of Deaf Children (ASDC)
Box 3355
Gettysburg
PA 17325
Phone- business - (Voice/TTY *(717) 334-7922*
Fax: *(717) 334 8808*
Website: www.deafchildren.org/
Provides support, encouragement and P.O. information to the families of deaf and hard of hearing children.

Deaf-Reach
3521 12th Street NE,
Washington, D.C. 20017
Phone (Voice/TTY): *(202) 832-6681*
Fax: *(202) 832-8454*
Website: www.deaf-reach.org
Formerly the National Health Care Foundation for the Deaf it aims to maximise self-sufficiency in deaf adults needing specialist support services.

The Family Village
(Website only) www.familyvillage.wisc.educ/
This a multi-information website of organisations providing specialised information and advice to families with deaf children.

Illinois Iowa Center for Independent Living
3708 11th St.,
PO Box 6156
Rock Island, IL 61231
Phone - business - (Voice/TTY) *309-793-0090*
Phone - Toll Free (Voice/TTY) *877-541-2505*
Fax: *309-283-0097*
Website: www.iicl.com
Provides regional information, advice and assistance to the deaf/hard of hearing community.

League for the Hard of Hearing
50 Broadway, 6th Floor,
New York,
New York 10004.
Phone (Voice): *917-305-7800*
Fax: *917-305-7999*
TTY: *971-305-7888*
Website: www.lhh.org
Founded in New York it provides hearing rehabilitation for people who are hard of hearing, deaf or deaf-blind, and their families.

League for the Hard of Hearing - Florida
2800 W. Oakland Park Blvd, Suite 306,
Oakland Park, FL 33311.
Phone: *954-731-7200*
Voice/TTY: *954-731-7208*
Direct TTY: *954-485-6336*
(details as for their New York office)

National Association of the Deaf
814 Thayer Avenue
Silver Spring
MD 20910-4500
Voice phone *301-587-1788*
TTY: *301-587-1789*
Fax: *301-587-1791*
Website: www.nad.org
Works towards making America a better place for all deaf and hard of hearing people through its staff, Board, members of various committees and its State Associations.

Self Help for Hard of Hearing People
7910 Woodmont Ave, Suite 1200
Bethesda
Maryland 20814

Voice phone:	*301-657-2248*
TTY:	*301-657-2249*
Fax:	*301-913-9413*

Website: www.hearingloss.org
Provides advice and information on hearing loss. It has a national support network of local chapters and state organisations working together for people who are hard of hearing and their families.

Texas Association of the Deaf
P.O. Box 450328
Garland,
Texas 75045-0328
Website: www.deaftexas.org (email addresses of contacts are given on their website)
Provides information and education on the various issues affecting the lives of the deaf and hard of hearing communities in the state of Texas.

Virginia Association for the Deaf
Website: www.vad.org (email addresses of Committee members obtained via their website)
Promotes, protects and preserves the rights and quality of life of deaf and hearing individuals in Virginia. It is a member of the National Association of the Deaf.

Virginia Department for the Deaf and Hard of Hearing
1602 Rolling Hills Dr, Suite 203
Richmond,
Virginia 23229-5012
Voice phone/TTY: *(804) 662-9502*
Voice phone/TTY (Toll free) (800) 552-7917
Website: www.vddhh.org
Works to reduce the communication barriers between those who are deaf or hard of hearing and their families and the professionals who serve them.

American Tinnitus Association
PO Box 5
Portland
OR 97207-0005
Phone (Toll Free within the U.S) *(800) 634-8978*
Phone (business) *(503) 248-9985*
Fax *(503) 248-0024*
Website: www.ata.org
Provides information and resources on tinnitus and hearing conservation.

Menières.Org
Website only: www.menieres.org
This website was founded to provide a 'home' of support for those who are suffering from Menière's Disease.

Canine Companions for Independence
P.O. Box 446
Santa Rosa,
CA 95402-0466
Phone (toll-free): *1-866-224-3647*
Website: www.caninecompanions.org
Provides highly-trained assistance dogs and ongoing support for people with disabilities. For full details of their work, regional sites and contacts visit their website.

Dogs for the Deaf, Inc.
10175 Wheeler Road
Central Point,
OR 97502
Voice phone/TDD: *541-826-9220*
Fax: *541-826-6696*
Website: www.dogsforthedeaf.org
Rescues unwanted dogs and professionally trains them to help hard of hearing people to lead more independent lives.

Florida Dog Guides For the Deaf (FTD), Inc.
P.O. Box 20662
Bradenton
FL 34203
Phone: (941) 748-8245
Website: www.dogguidesftd.org
Provides specially trained Dog Guides, including Hearing Dog Guides, to assist Florida's disabled members of the community.

International Hearing Dogs, Inc.
5901 E. 89th Avenue
Henderson
CO 80640
Voice phone/TDD: (303) 287-3277
Fax: (303) 287-3425
Website: www.members.aol.com/IHDI
Trains and places hearing dogs with adults who are deaf or hard-of-hearing, with and without multiple disabilities.

San Francisco SPCA
2500 16th Street
San Francisco
CA 94103-4213
Phone: (415) 554-3000
Fax: (415) 552-7041
Website: www.sfspca.org
Trains and places hearing dogs with deaf and hard of hearing adults residing in California and Nevada.